W9-AGE-584

THE

THIN

COMMANDMENTS

DIET

THE 10 NO-FAIL STRATEGIES
FOR PERMANENT WEIGHT LOSS

STEPHEN GULLO, Ph.D.

AUTHOR OF THIN TASTES BETTER

RODALE

Notice

This book is intended as a reference volume only, not as a medical manual. The information given here is designed to help you make informed decisions about your health. It is not intended as a substitute for any treatment that may have been prescribed by your doctor. If you suspect that you have a medical problem, we urge you to seek competent medical help.

Mention of specific companies, organizations, or authorities in this book does not imply endorsement by the publisher, nor does mention of specific companies, organizations, or authorities imply that they endorse this book.

Internet addresses and telephone numbers given in this book were accurate at the time it went to press.

© 2005 by Dietech Co.

All rights reserved. No part of this publication may be reproduced or transmitted in any form or by any means, electronic or mechanical, including photocopying, recording, or any other information storage and retrieval system, without the written permission of the publisher.

Printed in the United States of America
Rodale Inc. makes every effort to use acid-free ∞, recycled paper ♻.

Book design by Christina Gaugler

Library of Congress Cataloging-in-Publication Data

Gullo, Stephen P. (Stephen Pernice)
    The thin commandments diet : the 10 no-fail strategies for permanent weight loss / Stephen Gullo.
        p.   cm.
    Includes index.
    ISBN-13 978–1–57954–898–8 trade hardcover
    ISBN-10 1–57954–898–9 trade hardcover
    1. Reducing diets.   I. Title.
    RM222.2.G792   2005
    613.2'5—dc22   2004019995

Distributed to the trade by Holtzbrinck Publishers

    4   6   8   10   9   7   5   3   hardcover

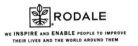

RODALE
WE INSPIRE AND ENABLE PEOPLE TO IMPROVE
THEIR LIVES AND THE WORLD AROUND THEM

FOR MORE OF OUR PRODUCTS
WWW.RODALESTORE.COM
(800) 848-4735

To Ruth Edelman

Indomitable advocate on behalf of mental health and humanitarian causes across America, leader in the civic life of the city of Chicago, who, along with her daughter, Renee Edelman, has been the greatest of friends and advisors. Thank you for being a true "guardian angel."

To Dr. Austin Kutscher

Distinguished professor in the department of psychiatry at Columbia University and president of the American Institute of Life-Threatening Illness at the Columbia-Presbyterian Medical Center, who has been my most inspiring teacher and mentor. Your pioneering work and monumental contributions to the sciences and health care have touched the lives of thousands and have profoundly shaped my professional life and all that I have done and will do in my career. I am forever grateful.

To my colleagues in nutrition, bariatric medicine, and dietetics

Who work each day on the front lines of weight control and who have contributed so much to the management of obesity and weight problems.

Contents

Acknowledgments

Many people have nurtured both my life and work, and I will always be grateful to them.

My family has loved and supported me unconditionally, and to my sisters, Angela Barna, Marianne Froelich, and Antoinette Pahlck; my nephews and nieces Christian and Karen Hanny and now little Kate Rose Hanny, Matthew Touron, and Maurene Levine; and my brothers-in-law, Joseph Barna, Allan Froelich, and Robert Pahlck, I say a profound *thank you*. I will always owe a special debt of gratitude to my sister Angela and my brother-in-law Joseph, who cared for my father so selflessly during his final illness.

I have been blessed with a loving second family in Mathew and Lee Love, along with Wendy and Lance Barnard and the late and beloved Florence Lazar-Galleau, who generously donated so much of her time and talents to help me as I started my career.

Along the road of my life, many friends have made enormous contributions to my growth: Dr. David and the late Marilyn Kohn, Drs. Daniel and Justine Carr, Duane Perez, Jason Capuano, Gloria Futterweit, Dr. Dan Cherico, Dr. Marc Shatz, Dr. Henry Berger, Anthony Abreu, Peter Swersey, John Contini, Anne Hearst, George Paxinos, Steve Zubkoff, Kent Keets, Douglas Kohn, Ronni Janoff-Weinstein and Barry Weinstein, Scott Yacker, Erica Morales, Dee Kerner, Mike Nelligan, Joanna Silverblatt, Luis Soto, and, of course, my dear friends and associates Edoardo Danilan and Nina Danilan. I am particularly grateful for the personal and professional support given to me and my work by my esteemed friends Jack Rudin, Leon Wagener, Gloria Milstein Flanzer, and Louis Flanzer. The rarest of human qualities is generosity of spirit and they are the definition of this spirit.

All that I have and will accomplish in my professional life would not be possible without the support of a gifted and dedicated team that assists me each day at the Institute for Health & Weight Sciences. Rosemarie Passaro has been with me from the very beginning, as a colleague and cherished friend, and her stewardship of our financial matters is so crucial. I will always be grateful to a remarkable man, her late husband, Tom Passaro. Norbert Bogner, my office manager and friend, oversees the daily operations and deals brilliantly with my often crazy schedule. Mike Nelligan is our "troubleshooter." He "makes it all happen." Mikhail Pomeranets skillfully assisted me with numerous aspects of this book and gave me and my writers invaluable guidance on computer matters.

At crucial points in my development, I was able to call on the wisdom of several professors and advisors who enhanced my life with their guidance: Dr. Rosalea Schonbar, late director of the clinical psychology program at Columbia University, Dr. David Peretz, the late Dr. B. Schoenberg, and Rev. Harold Robertson.

Two of my closest friends, Dr. Andrew Lassman and Lenin De La Cruz, have been constant sources of support and encouragement to me at each step in the writing of this book. Andrew is also a brilliant young scientist who gives me a forum to share and formulate scientific ideas. I thank both of them in these pages so they will know how much their support has meant to me. A top personal trainer and colleague, Brett Austin, contributed his scientific knowledge and insights to evaluating important research along with introducing me to the concept of volumizing.

Each week I call on the professional expertise of a group of gifted advisors: Dr. David Kohn, Hon. Michael Kalnick, and Nellon Chu. Their guidance has enabled me to navigate around so many of life's pitfalls. I also want to add a special word of thanks to a singularly talented litigator, Alan Green.

Miriam Rubin, a gifted, world-class chef, provided invaluable assistance with recipes and cooking skills, and Elissa Meadow, CEO and proprietor of Los Angeles's new Solar Harvest restaurant, was extraordinarily generous in contributing some of that restaurant's outstanding recipes.

Luis Soto, one of New York's premier trainers and life coaches, has helped many of my clients achieve their optimal potential and has been a wise and gifted advisor on exercise.

In recent years a number of outstanding people have entered my life and shared their friendship and expertise with me. Renee Edelman has always also been so generous with her time and expertise, and the success of *Thin Tastes Better* would never have been possible without Rene and her mother, Ruth Edelman. I also want to thank a brilliant journalist, George Christy, for his support. Both his pen and his intellect are a true gift to so many.

In the writing and marketing of this book, so many individuals gave invaluable guidance. Holly McCord, former nutrition editor at *Prevention* magazine, initially suggested to me that I bring this book to Rodale. Tami Booth, vice president, editor-in-chief of women's health books at Rodale, was the first person in publishing to read the proposal for this book and her appreciation for my work was a determining factor in selecting Rodale as my publisher. Tami introduced me to the team that would shape this work. Margot Schupf, executive editor, has guided me throughout the writing of this book with her insights and wisdom. Whenever I had a question or concern, Margot has always been there for me. Editor Christine Bucks has labored endlessly to edit this book and articulate its message. I am grateful for her important work, most of all her patience through all of my rewrites. I have found in the executive and professional staffs of Rodale gifted leaders and individuals who have supported and shaped this book: Amy Rhodes, vice president and publisher of trade books; Nancy Bailey, senior project editor; Cathy Gruhn, director of publicity, trade books; Cindy Ratzlaff, vice president of Rodale books; Dana Bacher, marketing director of trade books; Leslie Schneider, director of trade sales; and Sara Sellar, editorial assistant, women's health books, all of whom have been enormously helpful with their professional excellence. In a very real sense, I owe a unique debt to the Rodale family, for it was as a young boy reading *Prevention* magazine that my interest in health and health care first began.

I want to thank the prominent researchers and scientists whose pioneering work has been discussed in this book and who generously agreed to be interviewed: Dr. Virend K. Somers, professor of medicine in the division of cardiovascular disease and hypertension at the Mayo Clinic School of Medicine; Richard A. Anderson, Ph.D., lead scientist at the Beltsville Human Nutrition Research Center in Maryland; Michael Zemel, Ph.D., chairman of the nutrition department at the University of Tennessee; Dr. Sarah Leibowitz, professor at the Rockefeller University laboratory of behavioral neuroscience in New York City; C. Wayne Calloway, endocrinologist at George Washington University in Washington, D.C.; Linda Bartoshuk, professor of the Yale University School of Medicine; Valerie Duffy, Ph.D., assistant professor of dietetics at the University of Connecticut; and Dr. Walter Futterweit, clinical professor of medicine at Mount Sinai Medical School and chief, endocrine clinics, at Mt. Sinai—one of the nation's premier endocrinologists. Dr. Futterweit first introduced me to Polycystic Ovarian Syndrome and generously helped me to understand its implications for weight management. He is truly the consummate "doctors' doctor" and a great healer.

Robert Barnett, Esq., of Williams & Connolly, was the erudite and gifted attorney who made possible the sale of this book and who once again proved the wisdom of our mutual friends, Ruth and Daniel Edelman. I want to also thank Sylvia, Mr. Barnett's executive assistant, who "always gets it right."

No acknowledgments would be complete without thanking a great friend and author, Sugar Rautbord. Through her unmatched abilities to persuade and her honored position in the media community, she played a decisive role in the success of *Thin Tastes Better*. I will always be in her debt. Thank you, Sugar. You are the very best.

Carol Southern of Crown/Carol Southern Books was the gifted editor of my earlier work, *Thin Tastes Better*. That book would never have become a reality without her vision and support. The fact that it went on to become a national bestseller is a tribute to her leadership. Catherine Heusel-Grillo and Joseph Amodio were the most talented writers who made *Thin Tastes Better* possible. Catherine has become a friend I cherish deeply. It was she who crafted the organization and the writing of the proposal for this present book. She did so much to brilliantly take this book from concept to reality.

A team of gifted writers shaped this book and brought it to you. Each contributed unique talents.

Kathleen Quinn entered this project at a critical point and had to restart the project from scratch. She helped me enormously during a difficult period when I was recovering from an accident and also trying to write critical chapters. Her experience and talents as a seasoned journalist proved invaluable in writing the commandments, "Think Historically, Not Just Calorically," "Separate Mood from Food," and "Structure Gives Control." Lee Quarfoot, a distinguished editor and journalist, assisted me in the writing of the preface, the first commandment on strategy, "Box It In, Box It Out," and the commandment on deprivation. Lee has endlessly shared professional guidance with me throughout this project. She is the consummate professional. Jim Gerard, a highly experienced journalist who has taught journalism at the university level, did much of the research and writing for my seminal commandment, "The Problem May Be in the Food, Not in You," as well as contributing his talents to the writing and editing of other parts of the book. Bob Montgomery, a seasoned professional who has taught writing at one of the nation's leading universities, lent his considerable acumen and talents to "Treat Your Calories Like Dollars," and "Slips Should Teach You, Not Defeat You." Bob also edited and rewrote critical aspects of this book, for which I owe him a great deal of gratitude.

I would like to thank David Nayor, a gifted health journalist who made monumental contributions to this book and its readers. David did the painstaking research, interviewing, and nearly all the writing for the diet section and for "Losing Weight Is Half the Job, Keeping It Off Is the Other Half."

The Thin Commandments Diet is a tribute to the writing skills of these distinguished colleagues. I thank each of them.

On a personal note, I want to recognize a singular group of health professionals whose contributions to the advancement of medicine and the lives of their patients I admire greatly: Dr. Ben Lewis, Dr. Arnold Liscio, Dr. Jimmie Holland, Dr. David Peretz, Dr. Orli Etingin, Dr. Louis Aronne, Dr. Artemis Simopoulos, Dr. Eli Lizza, Dr. Daniel Carr, Dr. Jesse Rosenthal, Dr. Sheenah Hankin, and Dr. William Suozzi. I owe a particular debt of great gratitude to Dr. Daniel Baker, my friend and one of the world's preeminent plastic and reconstructive surgeons, who has helped me and so many others recover fully from the traumas of surgery for life-threatening illness. These individuals represent "the best of the best" of American medicine and health care.

My acknowledgments for this book could never fail to mention a group of people I hold in great esteem: my clients. They are a truly enlightened group of people who appreciate that, in the end, it is not just about dieting but self-mastery over self-regret. Among them stand many of the brightest and toughest intellects of American society, men and women who have made an outstanding contribution to our world through their exemplary personal lives, the families they have shaped, and their leadership in guiding preeminent universities, teaching hospitals, major corporations, and cultural and financial institutions. Some are fortunate enough to be the rich and famous and winners of Academy Awards and the prestigious prizes of the worlds of science and sports. But most are people just like you and me, who care deeply about the quality of their lives and who adamantly refuse to lose to a piece of food. They have been my greatest teachers, toughest reviewers, and most enthusiastic supporters for more than a quarter century.

Lastly, I have only one regret—that my late mother, Rose Pernice Gullo, is not here to see this book. Through her love and caring, she has shaped all that I have done and will do in my life. My gratitude and respect for this woman I was blessed to call "mother" is eternal.

Stephen Pernice Gullo
New York City
A.M.D.G.

Introduction

Calories are only half of the weight loss equation.

Now, welcome to the other half . . .

It has been said that the good doctor learns from his patients. My real education in the field of weight sciences began almost 25 years ago when I stopped looking at textbooks and prevailing theories for answers and starting *listening* to the men and women who came to me for help. It was only then that I realized why the standard approach to weight control was failing most people.

Earlier, as a student and then as a researcher and professor of human behavior and health sciences at the Columbia-Presbyterian Medical Center, I had learned that a thorough medical and personal history is critical to accurate diagnosis and identifying effective treatments. As I met with more and more clients, it became clear that the field of weight control was missing this guiding principle of health care. Indeed, *weight control may be the only area of health care where history—in this case, the patient's unique food history—is completely ignored.*

By looking *historically*—not just calorically—at my clients' dieting, weight loss, and weight gain, I saw that there were obstacles that repeatedly led these men and women down the path to failure. For some, it was a particular food. For some, it was a type of food, such as sweets or nibble foods. For others, it was a behavioral pattern, such as skipping meals or eating when they were bored or upset. When my patients incorporated new eating patterns, they would lose weight. When they returned to their old ways, control would be lost—and, like clockwork, the weight would come back. *They were gaining back the same weight with the same foods on the same days of the week at the same times over and over again. This was the one area of their lives where they were not learning from past mistakes!*

These individual patterns comprise what I call your Eating Print—the living history of the specific foods, situations, places, and responses that make up the mosaic of your unique eating behaviors. *Your Eating Print is your own unique signature in the world of food.* Just like our fingerprints, everyone's Eating Print has distinctive characteristics, and once you know your Eating Print, you can predict your behavior in any food situation, with any food. You can anticipate—and then prepare with strategy. Indeed, as I tell my own clients, once you know who you are in the world of food, you can predict how you will behave.

Unfortunately, every day millions of overweight Americans are given one-size-fits-all diets that directly contradict the lessons of their food history and Eating Prints. For example, the prevailing wisdom is that there are no good or bad foods. The statement is right, but the reasoning is wrong—*there are no good or bad foods; there are only good or bad histories with a food.* And *ignoring your personal history with such foods is what sets you up for failure.* It's quite simple: Those who violate their food history fail, and those who honor their food history succeed. In this book, I will help you to understand the power of knowing your Eating Print and how to use these lessons to dramatically increase your success. I will teach you the critical concept that has changed my clients' approach to dieting forever. *When it comes to evaluating a food and its value for your weight control, think historically, not just calorically!* You will learn why history comes before calories in determining a food's suitability for your success at weight control.

When you break with the philosophy of dieting that thinks of calories alone and start to think historically, you individualize the world of food to your own past habits and unique eating patterns. The question, "What is my history with this food (or this type of food)?" is a powerful mechanism to evaluate any food and a way to discover whether it will work for your success or against it. This fundamental shift in your thinking will change your perspective on the world of food forever. It is a shift that all my winners at weight control have made. We cannot possibly address in this book every food you have or will encounter, but once you make this shift in your thinking, you will have what I call "the North Star" to guide you.

Diets succeed because they give structure to out-of-control eating and impose limits on foods. But once the diet is over, the boundaries are lifted and the limits are removed, sending people with weight problems out into the world with nothing but general guidelines on the importance of a "balanced diet" and standard advice on enjoying their favorite foods "in moderation." This advice ignores the obvious fact: that those who can eat moderately would not need a diet in the first place. Indeed, it's counter to the lessons of human history that in manners of pleasure and passion human beings are not given to moderation, but to excess. Can we really be surprised that so many people gain weight back?

If I could make one contribution to the field of weight control, it would be to make the field pay attention to food history. How can you expect a person to magically control a food or behavior that's been out of control for decades? It's not enough to recommend moderation. You have to study that person's history and give them the skills to control what their history has shown to be problem areas.

THE OTHER HALF OF THE EQUATION . . .

Since its inception, the multibillion dollar weight loss industry has been dominated by scores of experts who have counseled overweight people on what to eat and what not to eat. A single common focus has linked virtually every diet program ever developed: an emphasis on calories, balancing them, limiting them, and trying to burn them off. But I have broken away from this prevailing approach and have developed an entirely new paradigm for weight control—a paradigm *that emphasizes history before calories and replaces willpower with strategy—strategies that transform struggle into success. For strategy is stronger than willpower. It is this that makes success not only possible, but easy.* And unlike many weight programs, the techniques and skills of the food strategy approach are truly universal, whether you're doing it alone, working with a nutritionist or dietitian, or following a commercial diet program—from high protein/low carbohydrate regimes like the Atkins Diet, to structured plans like Weight Watchers or Jenny Craig. This is the first weight control book to prove that—*with the right strategies—anyone can successfully manage their weight and make the fundamental shift from dieter to food strategist.*

The deeper I delved into my clients' histories, the clearer it became that it would take far more than nutritional advice and behavior modification to conquer their strong social, biological, and psychological programming. The traditional approach to weight control can't possibly address all these variables. In fact, it addresses only one—food and its calories.

A generation ago, perhaps, this model met a crying need. Our grandparents didn't understand the complexities of calories, carbohydrates, cholesterol, and fats. But today we know which foods are good for our bodies and which foods undermine our health. *The problem facing this generation is not calories alone, but control.* That is why so many diet programs fail. They focus almost exclusively on calorie management, while ignoring the destructive food programming of a lifetime. However, the purpose of this book is not just to share with you the best eating plan for safe and rapid weight loss or the 10 most crucial skills for success in weight control. It's about what few, if any, weight programs have ever dealt with: how to change your fundamental thoughts and feelings about the very foods that have created your weight problem, so you're not always struggling with feelings of deprivation. If you're reading these words, chances are that you have lost weight many times, but you have never once changed your thinking about food.

But you have not been failing. Dieting has been failing you, by neglecting to teach you the strategies that you need to succeed. Without these, every one of your attempts at weight loss has been and will continue to be an unending struggle with willpower.

The 10 Percent Solution

The strategies that I will teach you in this book are not my own. They have been taught to me by the most powerful of all teachers—the thousands of my clients who have succeeded at weight control. They will help you not only to lose weight but also to change your thinking, so that you'll feel that you—not a cookie or a breadbasket—are calling the shots.

In *The Thin Commandments Diet,* I have distilled decades of my work and the lessons of the winners at weight control into the 10 most critical strategies for success at weight loss and the unique diet that makes it possible . . . and enjoyable.

Because of my early training in developmental and motivational psychology, my instinct has always been to focus on an individual's strengths rather than weaknesses. Early in my career, as I contemplated my clients' dilemmas, my thoughts turned to the minority of people who *do* succeed at weight loss not only for the duration of their diet but also for years afterward. While success is defined differently in different studies—many use a low standard of keeping off just 5 pounds for only one year, which in my opinion isn't enough to define a lifestyle—the research with stringent standards suggests that somewhere between 3 and 10 percent of dieters who manage to lose a significant amount of weight (at least 10 to 100 pounds) keep it off for five years or more.

For this elusive group—the real winners of weight loss—thin endures. I wondered what it is that they do that keeps them from becoming part of the 90 percent or more who lose weight only to gain it back? And how could I use these insights to help those caught in the pattern of yo-yo dieting? *What is the 10 percent solution?*

The answers to these questions are the message of *The Thin Commandments Diet.*

Advertising Empowers Dieting

From the very start of my graduate studies, I have been fascinated by the motivational techniques of the advertising world and their power to change behavior. Every day, advertisers convince millions of people to part with their money and to feel privileged. They reverse centuries of practical financial programming handed down to us through American history, since the era of Benjamin Franklin (i.e., a penny saved is a penny earned), and lure us into buying things—expensive cars, designer sneakers—for which we often have little if any need.

These campaigns succeed because they plant a new internal language and belief system in people who otherwise might not even care about the product. By repeating certain key ideas and slogans again and again, they instill a message; creating a very real and enduring psychological need for the advertiser's products. Sound familiar? "Just do it," and "I'll bet you can't eat just one." No matter what the product may be, advertisers create a need for it that is so strong that it overrides another need—the need for money.

Food advertisers teach the very same lesson—that the smell, feel, and taste of their foods are so compelling we need to have them, regardless of their cost to our health, looks, and self-esteem.

I realized this same technique could be harnessed to overcome decades of food programming and could be used to motivate dieters to succeed.

In the months and years that followed this revelation, I began adapting the tools of advertising to the world of weight control and created a technique called *cognitive switching* (which I fully explain on page 117) and an allied strategy called *mental rehearsal* (discussed on page 119) to help my clients prepare in advance for any food situation. By employing these powerful techniques, they could even desensitize themselves to the allure of tempting foods and eliminate the cravings and feelings of deprivation.

I studied how dieters talk to themselves about food and identified key phrases that form the core of their "food speak"—talk that creates a powerful need to eat certain foods and stirs up cravings and feeling of deprivation if they're not consumed. I created and taught my clients a new script that replaced the old "food speak" and showed them a new way to think about food. Through cognitive switching and mental rehearsal, simple techniques that you will soon master, my clients learned a new language and new way to become winners at weight control! They were empowered to put their need to be trim and look good before their need for food—even the foods that had sabotaged all their previous weight control efforts.

The Best Diet

Historically, one of the most frequently heard complaints is that diet program foods don't taste good. In 2005, that is a complete myth, especially in view of the world of food we now inhabit. In the decade since I wrote my first book, *Thin Tastes Better*, the whole universe of food has changed. We're now living in a veritable paradise that includes scrumptious low-fat cold cuts; gourmet Belgian waffles that pack less than 100 calories a serving; a miracle cracker that kills appetite yet contains only 16 calories; and a luscious chocolate truffle that's a mere 30 calories and rivals the best chocolates in Europe. Supermarkets, health food stores, and gourmet food shops across the country now stock diet products that can give you all the taste you want . . . without the calories. When you know these foods, you can enjoy your fill and never feel deprived . . . for dieting is no longer about deprivation but substitution. In Part 2, I identify the best of the best light foods, my Taste Is King award winners (see page 294). Time and time again, clients have told me that their success would have been impossible without these delicious substitutes, the diet foods that made success at weight control a pleasure instead of a struggle. Most significant, through the quick and easy recipes of my world class chefs, you'll enjoy 5-star dining without the calories.

It is the only diet program in the world designed not only on the basis of calories, carbs, and grams of fat but also around *your* behavior and food preferences. It teaches you not only which are the best foods for weight loss but also how to predict which foods are most likely to sabotage your success. Now you can select foods on the basis of calories and your ability to succeed on this diet. And through the vehicle of the unique "new scale," *you will have the only tool in the world of weight control that can predict which of your day-to-day behaviors are early warning signs of problems ahead and how to quickly avoid them.*

The strategies I'm about to share with you have been featured in over 20 national and international cover stories, including a *New York Times* Lifestyle section article that recognized my success rate as far surpassing any known standards in the diet industry. Through the pages of this book, you will learn the eating plan and unique strategies for which my clients have paid $1,000 an hour and waited up to a year for an appointment. Perhaps this is one of the greatest testimonies to the power and effectiveness of what you will read herein.

Unlike diet books that just tell you about what works to lose weight, I will also tell you about what works for the psyche, what makes it easy to stay with this diet, and what works for real people who live life on the go. *The Thin Commandments Diet is the missing link in the gap between knowing what to do and knowing how to do it.* For those who struggled with their weight, it's the key that can unlock the door to permanent weight loss.

In this book, I will take you through these simple strategies step-by-step, guiding you along the path that has brought so many people to their personal, permanent thin. Through the use of these creative and winner-tested strategies, you will learn to do things in a new way—an easier way—and get a new result: success.

No matter how many times you failed in the past, and regardless of all the setbacks, remember that you have never given up. You have always held on to that desire for success. And how strong and powerful that desire must be! You and I together "will find a way, or make one." I have seen it work for thousands of people; *for dieting is about losing weight. . . food strategy is about ending the problem!*

BEYOND DIETING: YOUR LIFE FACTOR

I want you to think about why you bought this book. It wasn't just to read words on a page, learn my philosophy of weight control, or even fit into your clothes. On the most fundamental level, you bought this book because there was a discomfort or unhappiness in your life. An unhappiness with your weight, your appearance, the fit of your clothes, the amount of control food exercised over you, and the way you were dealing with it. Through these pages, you will find the path to remove this unhappiness and in its place improve your appearance and enhance your health and the quality of your life. This is the blessing that you will give to yourself.

To eat according to the principles of this book is not about dieting; it's about being food-smart and life-smart. It takes dieting out of the old association with deprivation and puts it into the larger context of your life. It is about the quality of your life—looking younger and living longer, at the top of your game.

This book is, in the end, about empowerment, and that most elusive of all human goals—happiness.

I joke with my clients that when I'm 80 and in God's waiting room, when everyone else is taking the Prozac of the day, I'll be making the rounds of all the pizzerias and bakeries. In fact, I plan to leave this world in a pizza truck!

In the meantime, none of us wants to look back to the prime of our lives when we had our youthfulness, attractiveness, and health and realize that we squandered it all to hang out with a bread basket, a bag of candies, or a pizza pie. This is the greatest deprivation of all.

There's a powerful line in Elton John and Tim Rice's Broadway hit, *Aida*: "We are given paradise, but only for a day." And though our lives aren't paradise, we have the power and the privilege to make them better and to appreciate what is truly meaningful and eternal. This is our "day."

In the end, you must face the truth: You have seen and tasted it all in the world of food. It has not made you happy; it has only made you heavy. There has got to be a better way. This book is the better way.

PART I

THE THIN COMMANDMENTS

The First Thin Commandment:
Strategy Is Stronger Than Willpower

COMMANDMENT ESSENTIALS

- Use strategy to stay in control.
- Stop self-defeating food talk.
- Weigh yourself on the New Scale for Dieting.
- Keep a food diary.
- Listen to a power tape.

THE SINGLE GREATEST SURPRISE of my professional life has been the discovery that success at weight control is *not* about willpower. Indeed, those who succeed at weight control do not have greater willpower than those who fail—they just have better strategies. This is the most powerful lesson I have learned in 25 years from almost 15,000 clients.

Like you—and many of my colleagues—I once had quite a few preconceptions about people with weight problems: They lack willpower to control their eating; they have psychological or emotional issues that keep them from permanently losing weight; and they lack the food smarts to follow a healthy diet.

When I actually began to work with these individuals, I discovered that almost all of my preconceptions were wrong. They were successful in their professional lives, enjoyed many interests, and had meaningful personal relationships. They were creative people with vision, who cared passionately about their goals and were dedicated to excellence. They epitomized the American ideal of determination and success.

Far from lacking nutritional knowledge, many of my clients already knew *what* to eat and what *not* to eat. They'd read diet book after diet book, were aware of calories, carbohydrates, and fats, and knew how to read labels. Many had lost hundreds of pounds over the years. But despite all their knowledge and weight loss, they had never been able to keep the pounds off permanently.

I struggled to reconcile my clients' success in every other area of their lives with their failure at weight control. How could these people—many of whom had overcome tremendous obstacles to achieve greatness—still lose control with chocolates or a breadbasket? They knew what they had to do to lose weight, but they were living in misery because they couldn't do it. Such repeated failure takes a terrible toll, even on the most successful individual.

WHY WE FAIL

By looking back across the years at my clients' dieting, weight loss, and gain, I've seen that *there are distinct and predictable patterns of behavior and food choices that have led these men and women to failure.* I have conclusively discovered that the particular diet an individual follows is secondary to success at weight control, which is why people can so easily switch diets from year to year. The most important factor for winning is having strategies—not the particular diet you follow.

In a recent article "The Diet That Works" in the *Wall Street Journal,* Tara Parker Pope captured the truth that resonates for a large number of individuals who struggle with weight control. "If sticking to a diet were easy, so many of us wouldn't be so fat."

The men and women who *have* avoided a weight problem—or conquered one on their own—instinctively use strategy to stay in control. It's the common thread that unites everyone who has ever won at weight control, including myself. Food strategy has saved me again and again in my own life.

Obviously, no one who has lost weight intends to gain it back. After every diet, every one of my clients was completely committed to maintaining his or her weight loss. But the commitment was overcome by a combination of powerful forces: biology, our value system, and advertising.

Recent research shows that our ancestors passed on powerful biological programming that may predispose us to crave and seek out certain foods, as many of us who are sensitive to sweet, salty, and bitter tastes know well. *These differences in sensitivity, not willpower, may explain why some people are able to maintain control around certain foods— such as chocolate chip cookies—while others find that these foods actually trigger increased appetite and losses of control.*

And unlike many of our ancestors, who had to struggle to find food, we are literally surrounded by it. Yet we still carry the ancestral mindset of "waste not, want not" in our modern society where food is overly abundant and always present. Just consider all of the food stores, fast-food chains, airport and shopping mall food courts—many of them open 24 hours a day! Overconsumption is the name of the game, and "all-you-can-eat" has become a national mantra. We have been steadily programmed to believe that it is our birthright to eat whatever we want, whenever we want. We're also bombarded by slick commercials that reinforce the belief that foods are the goodies and treats that make life worthwhile and wash away stress—and that any limitation of them is a horrible deprivation. Even the language of love is expressed in terms of food—honey, cookie, peaches, sweetie. And when you fall out of love, that person becomes a crumb!

Saddled with this powerful psychological and biological programming, surrounded by messages that food is the answer to every problem and the reward for every success, it's no wonder so many people fall back into the habits that lead to weight gain. And it's totally clear why so many feel instantly deprived when they think about weight control.

STRATEGY: THE KEY PRINCIPLES

Food situations are a part of every life. They come up again and again, and there's an amazing amount of predictability to what you can expect to encounter. Most of us rely on a very small assortment of foods—the same vegetables, the same meats, the same snack foods that satisfy an eat-and-run diet. Despite the fact that we can buy practically any food at any time, no matter how exotic or out of season, few of us venture beyond the limits of our favorite foods. And most eating occurs in only about seven situations: at home, in the workplace, in restaurants, in others' homes, when traveling, on vacation, and at celebratory events, such as holiday dinners, weddings, and parties. *The realm of food is not a big world, but a small village.*

The same scenarios come up over and over again. You face the same foods, the same temptations. However overwhelmed you may feel in the land of abundance, there is another more powerful truth at work as well: You have seen it all and tasted it all before. It may come in different shapes, varieties, and new presentations, but there's very little that's new in the world of food that you will face today. I will teach you strategies to deal with each situation. And I'll show you ways to develop your skills so that your responses become automatic. Rather than a constant tug-of-war that drains your willpower and resolve, you will have a set of tools to rely on, no matter where you go or what foods you may meet along the way.

Although food strategies vary depending on the person, the techniques share common themes. This chapter and those that follow will teach you a new way of dealing with your weight that involves key principles that have enabled so many of my clients to turn a lifetime of failure with weight into a lifetime of success.

• **Food history.** In a world of thousands of types of food, my careful research has revealed that only a handful are at the root of most weight problems. Food history shows that weight control is not a mountain to climb, just a few patterns to master.

• **Food desensitizing.** Techniques to defuse the power of cravings so that you can be around food that would normally tempt you without feeling deprived.

• **Breaking through food "baby talk."** Methods to transform self-defeating food talk learned in childhood—that can rule and ruin adulthood—into a new script, with phrases, thoughts, and values that work in the real world and prove that anyone can overcome feelings of deprivation.

- **The New Scale for Dieting.** A unique and effective tool for measuring the shifts and changes in your attitudes, skills, and motivation that can result in increased pounds, to be used as an early warning system *before* you step on a real scale. *The New Scale for Dieting predicts in advance if you'll be gaining weight* and makes it possible to prevent the seven most critical mistakes that lead to weight gain. This has never before been done in a weight program.

- **Containment.** The powerful technique that turns slips into success and teaches you how to cut off an error and never again feel the guilt of "I blew it."

- **Keeping the pleasure of food.** Enjoying favorite foods and not feeling deprived is critical for your success. Through recipes and food preparation techniques in my diet plan, you'll discover how to preserve the joy of eating without excess calories, and you will learn the best of the best of the new light foods, which my clients and I have tasted for you. Of the thousands of products we've sampled, only a handful have merited our Taste Is King award (see page 294). And the gourmet recipes will prove that success at weight control is not about giving up the pleasure of fine dining. Indeed, *not* to enjoy the foods on a weight plan guarantees failure!

Whenever I teach new clients the techniques for weight control, I know that I am training them for "diet fitness." For, just as you can become physically fit and train for a sport, every overweight person has the ability to become psychologically fit and train for long-term weight control. These strategies, along with many others that I will teach you, make it possible not only to dramatically increase your likelihood for success on a diet but also to maintain that success for years.

Some of these strategies may seem unusual or contradict what you have been led to believe about dieting and weight control. But successful weight control is not about doing what's "normal"—it's about doing what works for you. You should not be concerned about the norm—that's the preoccupation of the insecure—but about what brings you the success you deserve. As Chairman Deng responded when criticized by the Communist hardliners for introducing capitalist initiatives into China, "It doesn't matter if the cat is black or white; it only matters if it can catch mice."

DIETS ARE JUST WORDS ON A PAGE

Most of the diet books out there today focus on only half the equation: the right foods. *But that leaves out the most critical element for success—you!* Diets are just words on a page, a list on paper of what to eat. They don't help you plan what to think or say, and they don't tell you how to *behave*. They ignore the right behaviors, the critical issues of how to stay motivated and how to bounce back from a lapse, and how to avoid cravings and feelings of deprivation, and they don't change your thinking about food.

Strategy deals with how to make weight control easy. The right techniques actually encourage you to *want* to continue. They lead you to a way of eating that makes you feel happier and brings about permanent results by changing your mindset. At the core of the lessons I teach is changing the food programming that you've been taught since childhood.

The Lure of Food "Baby Talk"

When faced with cravings and feelings of deprivation, most dieters slide straight back into childhood—and that language that goes with it. "But it's my favorite." "It's not fair that I can't have it." "But I've been so good." "It's my comfort." "It's my treat." "I'll reward myself." This food "baby talk" is at the heart of many people's weight problems, drowning out their common sense and even their desire for health and sometimes life itself.

For many of my clients, this is the only area in their lives still run by the childhood patterns of thinking and conditioning. Indeed, for so many of us, it is the single area of living where childhood thinking has never been updated. *Where food is concerned, even the most mature adults often act like children—like children who want their way no matter what, blocking out the negative consequences of their eating.* They focus instead on a few minutes' worth of taste that fills the mouth and lingers for a short while, while completely denying the obvious and discomforting cost.

For these foods are not free—you have to wear them for years to come. You can't eat it all and still be thin. This is a fact. But you can be a selective gourmet and never have to give up the pleasure of fine dining.

Food is everywhere, and because it so often looks and tastes great, it's easy for us to continue to live in this childish mindset, telling ourselves "these are my goodies and treats." And we often listen to the message—until it creates disaster. The challenge is that the food is immediate, but the cost is often paid on the "layaway" plan. And like most layaway plans, the interest is high. Perhaps you have only to look in the mirror?

Only children live their lives believing they can have it all without any cost. Now it's time for you to bring this part of your life into the adult world. All of life contains adjustments and trade-offs. In accepting this, you not only establish a framework for lasting solutions to your weight problem, but you become a more resilient and mature human being. *It's time to stop resenting what you do to keep your body healthy and attractive.* Everything you value in your life—your relationships, your children, and your career—has taken work, focus, and endurance. Why should it be any different when it comes to managing your weight? Strategy, however, minimizes the cost and maximizes the reward.

The winners have come to this realization, and they no longer feel deprived, but liberated. In a recent survey of my clients, 86 percent said they felt no sense of deprivation. Without taking this step of growth and maturation, there can be no permanent weight loss, no permanent freedom. They've taken a turn in their evolution—evolving from childhood thinking and values into the adult thinking in the world of foods.

If you've come this far, you are already well on your way to that understanding and sense of freedom. You bought this book because you want to lose weight, and you want to do better at ongoing weight control. Now the choice to act is yours.

THREE SIMPLE STEPS

There are three actions that can encourage your progress, guard it, and enhance it. For thousands of my clients, these have proven to be among the most effective weapons available for arming themselves in their battle with weight. They reinforce all of the messages of this book, and I encourage you to do all three of them.

Weigh Yourself on the New Scale for Dieting

Scales don't keep people thin. Every heavy person owns a scale. The scale is the measure of pounds that tells us just how far we've strayed from thin. The regular scale is the end result of your behaviors; it reports where you have stood with the foods in your life since you last weighed in. The New Scale for Dieting predicts in advance which direction the regular scale will be moving—it provides an early warning system. The New Scale for Dieting is a simple 10-question quiz (see the opposite page) that reviews the basic skills and attitudes that you should be maintaining as part of your healthy life of thin. With it, you can track changes in your control skills and thinking in the same way that a diabetic tracks blood sugar or someone with hypertension monitors blood pressure. With regular use, it can alert you to areas where you may be weak and therefore vulnerable to slip-ups and bring your behavior and thinking in line with the winners at weight control. *The questions reflect the actions of those who succeed at weight control. In weighing yourself on the New Scale for Dieting, you have an instant means of knowing that you are on the same path.* I tell my clients to weigh themselves once a week on a regular scale and once a week on the New Scale for Dieting. This is to guide you to your goal. Once you reach your maintenance level, and the regular scale is no longer going down every week, your motivation will change, and you'll need another, modified New Scale (you'll find it on page 162) to use for quizzing yourself regularly, to protect all that you've accomplished.

Keep a Food Diary

In the studies on weight control, one factor keeps recurring: *Those who maintain a written record of what they're eating each day lose more weight and do significantly better at keeping it off than those who do not.* A food diary that tracks what and when you eat will allow you to detect any problems in your eating plan as they occur and to accurately gauge how much you are consuming. There is nothing else you can do that takes just a few minutes a day that will increase your weight loss and the likelihood of success as much as this.

I recommend keeping your food diary in a notebook beside your bed, where you can record in it, morning and night. Write down everything you eat, including any nibbles. To help identify your patterns, circle your errors: foods that you may have eaten in excessive amounts, foods not on your eating plan, and foods with hidden calories, such as those cooked in oil, butter, or sauces.

You might also find that it gives you an extra edge to plan meals in advance. You'll benefit from writing out the next day's menus

The New Scale for Dieting

Give yourself this quiz about once a week. If you're falling back into old patterns and an old foodie belief system, this exercise will make you aware of it. The commandments in this book are designed to help you ace the questions. Every time you ask them, your psyche gets the message about the behaviors and thinking that are becoming a natural part of your new lifestyle.

1. Am I going more than 3 to 4 hours without a healthy snack or meal?
2. Am I failing to plan (i.e., letting supplies of healthy foods run out, going into food situations hungry, failing to prepare for high-risk food situations, and failing to carry my ThinPack when traveling or going out for a busy day)? (See Chapter 4 for more on ThinPacks.)
3. Am I avoiding foods I have a long history of abusing?
4. Am I keeping my moods out of my foods? Am I not eating out of boredom or anger, and am I re-

minding myself in stressful situations that "this is not about food"?
5. Am I keeping problem foods out of the house or out of sight?
6. Am I avoiding high-risk situations (i.e., reading dessert menus, looking at dessert carts, dining in restaurants with buffet-style and/or family-style service)?
7. Am I maintaining finger control? Avoiding mindless nibbling?
8. Am I eating too much of the "right foods" (such as chicken or fruit) on my plan?
9. Am I watching for the hidden calories that stop weight loss (such as those found in salad dressings, foods made in butter or oil, sauces on food, and side dishes), and failing to ask in restaurants "what does it come with?" and "how's it prepared?"
10. Am I reminding myself that this is not about deprivation but doing what works for a happier, healthier life?

and snacks—especially if it's a day when you expect to be stressed out or to face an array of food temptations, or if you've seen some recent slippage and need to get back on the right footing and follow through. The advance notice programs the psyche and structures behavior. It works like an early fire-alarm system.

Listen to a Power Tape

Would you like to get the same training that my clients receive without paying thousands of dollars? Would you like to get the same benefits?

Making a recording, in any way that suits your lifestyle—on a cassette, CD, or any other electronic means—and listening to it frequently utilizes one of the most powerful techniques that I have adapted from the advertising world—that is, to reinforce a message by repeating certain key ideas and phrases again and again. It's a powerful tool not only for your behavior but for changing your lifelong thinking and feeling about food. As an instrument for weight control, it will push your buttons to motivate the behavior you want and extinguish the behavior you don't want. As you read this book, pick out several of the commandments—or go for all of them—to use in making tapes for yourself.

A food-control cassette is one of the surefire ways to quell cravings, short-circuit a sense of deprivation, and reinforce motivation and commitment. Basically, your tapes are an advertising campaign for you, and the product they are pitching is a new you. And like any successful ad campaign, they need to be upbeat, catchy, and full of powerful images that will capture your imagination and interest. In this chapter and the ones that follow, I've given you tips for writing your own scripts and three sample dialogues to help you through the three most critical moments in weight control:

1. Getting started

2. Keeping your motivation high, especially once you pass the midpoint of your weight loss, and you're starting to look and feel better

3. Adjusting to the lifestyle for maintenance

As you listen to the tapes regularly, your mind will absorb the message and start reinforcing it on its own, and your thought patterns will begin to mimic the ideas on the tapes. After just a few weeks of daily listening, you should begin to hear the words of your new food talk spontaneously. The repetition will begin to become your internal self-talk, and the changes will be seen not only in your attitude but also in your behavior with food.

Your cassette or CD is a cheerleader in your pocket, always there to give support. You can listen to it in your car on your way to work, or in the bathroom while you shave or shower in the morning, or while power walking around the neighborhood. You can draw on the tape at any time to help drown out the old food talk and reinforce your new inner dialogue.

Your recordings should be as unique and individual as you are. The scripts should be tailored to suit your own situation. You may find it more powerful to speak in the first person, saying, "I will start living today as I never have before!" Or, if a coaching tone works better for you, you might consider using the second-person: "*You* will start your food-control program today!" Write your scripts to accommodate your needs.

Once you have your library of food talk tapes, make sure you listen to them every day. While you're losing weight and even after you've reached your goal, don't stop tuning in. You don't have to listen every day, but don't cut them out completely. The biggest threat to your weight control is to get cocky and think you're cured. Thin is a lifestyle—not some arbitrary number on a scale. Remember, *you lose the weight; you don't lose the vulnerability.*

Play It Again . . . and Again . . . and Again

A food diary and a food-control recording are among the strongest weapons you have in your weight-loss arsenal, a frontline defense in the battle for control over your body. Don't underestimate their power. Writing a message *and* hearing a message over and over again sinks that message indelibly into your conscious and subconscious mind. The tapes are designed to drown out the old messages that food is sending you—"I have to have it. It looks so delicious. It's so interesting."—and to empower you and keep you focused in challenging situations, such as when you're under stress or bored.

(continued on page 16)

Sample Tape #1: Getting Started

Make listening to a tape a regular part of your routine. Hearing the messages in the morning can be especially effective, getting you off on the right foot to face the day and follow through. This script will help to get you started. Edit it however it suits you to address your vulnerabilities and reprogram your thinking.

You may feel a bit awkward at first as you speak into the tape recorder. But like so many aspects of food control, the consistent and faithful repetition of the process makes it easier and easier to do.

- "What is wrong with this picture of my life that I am losing to a piece of food, taking orders from a cookie (or whatever your problem foods may be)?"
- "I will start my food plan today. I don't want to wait. I won't say that I'll start eating well tomorrow. How many times have I said that before? Saying tomorrow is saying I will *not* do it today. *This* is the tomorrow I spoke of yesterday. I would never run a business the way I've treated my own body and my weight problem. If this were something that I needed to do for my children or someone I love, I would have done it a long time ago. Now, indeed, I will do

it for someone I love—myself."
- "Today, I'll start living as never before. I'll remember that thin begins in the supermarket. I will buy the foods that support my success and avoid the ones that sabotage it. If I don't buy it, I don't eat it. If it's not in my kitchen, it's not on my hips."
- Remind yourself why you're doing this. "None of my clothes fit. I can't bear to look at a picture of myself or in the mirror. I'm not taking care of my health or the quality of my life."
- Talk about the journey. "There's not a single food that I'll see today that I haven't seen or tasted before. I have seen it all, I've tasted it all, and it hasn't made me happy; it has only made me heavy. This is not a mountain to climb. It is just a few patterns to master. I have overcome a great deal in my life. I can learn to manage three meals and two or three snacks a day. That is my only challenge to buy a lifetime of being trim. What's the worst that can happen to me? I will just see or smell a food that I'd like to eat. It will not be new. I have seen and tasted it before. A food temptation is simply a feeling, it's not a command. It lasts about 4 to 12 min-

utes. If I break the eye contact and say 'No way!' it will pass. Isn't thin worth 4 to 12 minutes of standing up to a feeling?"

- Remind yourself of your history. "What I have done in the past has not worked. That's why I will do it a new way using strategy. If it seemed difficult in the past, it probably was because I didn't have strategy. I knew what I wanted—to be trim— but I didn't have a plan to get there and stay there. Strategy gives me the road map that makes it possible. It's not just knowing what to eat and what not to eat. It's knowing how to do it, how to want to do it, and how to make it easy to do. That's what strategy is about, and that's what I'm working on, one day at a time."

- Focus on the foods and the habits that have contributed to your weight problem. Name your problem foods and problem behaviors. If you've decided that certain foods have made you fail repeatedly, and you want to avoid them while you're trying to lose weight, be very clear and strong with yourself. Either say you are going to temporarily eliminate these foods from your life, or you are going to limit them to special situations. If you've

decided to limit specific foods by reserving them for certain times or places, say to yourself, "I will only eat them on the weekend . . . or Sunday night . . . never in a restaurant and never at home."

- If you are a stress eater, be sure to remind yourself that food doesn't solve problems. "If I have an upsetting situation, I will say to myself, I have an uncomfortable feeling, but it is not about food. Eating over it will not make me happy; it will only make me heavy. Even if I can't solve the problem or change the person who is upsetting me, by not eating, I break a major pattern that has made me heavy. Maybe I can't do anything about other problems in my life, but my weight is one area that I have the power to change. And I will use that power."

- End with empowerment and perspective. "In a world where there is cancer, and AIDS, and homelessness, what's the big deal if I say no thanks to (problem food), so I can say yes to being thin? Did I come this far in life to take orders from a (problem food)? Remind yourself of your power. I deserve to be trim. I deserve to succeed with this. I deserve to be in control in my life with food."

The diary and tapes can keep you from falling into the pattern of doing what you've always done.

Repetition is one of the most powerful tools of advertising. Throughout this book, I'll be repeating key phrases over and over again. This is by intent, to help you change your thinking, not just to have you read words and forget them. Together, we'll use techniques to enhance your life and sell you on a new, thin, all-you-can-be you!

DISCOVER WHERE YOU STAND

Weight loss, like most things in life, occurs in stages, over time. Different thoughts, emotions, and levels of motivation mark each stage. For most dieters, feelings of ambivalence and indecisiveness toward old food temptations start to surface after a while. You may diet for many weeks without a hint of a doubt, untroubled by any seductive signals from favorite foods or old eating habits. But then you can begin to waver.

More than likely, you've reached one of the critical, problematic spots of dieting. To maintain your weight—and your control over food—you need to be aware of where you stand in this progression of stages. When you truly know who you are, where you are, and how you perform in the world of food, you can predict how you will behave—and, if necessary, take steps to remain on track and to bolster your flagging motivation and confidence.

Sometimes, after an initial rapid weight loss, the pound drop starts to slow, and you can become discouraged. That's the time to recall that your new program isn't just about losing pounds, it's about losing the problem of yo-yo dieting. Another danger is that, sometimes, after the weight starts to come off, and the clothes get loose, you may develop the misconception that you are already thin, when, in fact, you are simply a little less overweight. The truth is, it's easy to delude yourself, to think because your weight is less, your vulnerability is less, and your need for the strategies is less. On the contrary, strategy becomes more important as a dieter progresses through the phases, and it is most critical in the final phase of maintenance.

Losing weight doesn't change your history, your taste buds, or your vulnerability, so it's essential to avoid becoming sloppy with the strategies or the planning—that's the first critical lesson to master: *Think strategy.*

The Three Most Critical Points in a Diet Plan

In working with my clients, I've found three stages in the process of weight control that pose the greatest risk of derailing a weight program and undermining a new eating lifestyle. Navigating through these challenges is the path to truly mastering your control with food.

• **At the beginning.** The motivation to start dieting often begins with a desire to look better, to fit into your clothes, to feel better about yourself, and to improve your health—and it often means experiencing strong, very negative feelings. You may feel disgusted with yourself for your lack of control, or hate to look at yourself in the mirror, or dread opening your closet in the morning because you have nothing to wear that will make you feel good about yourself. Although this is the stage that propels many overweight people into treatment, it can also become a black hole, in which motivation to change is overwhelmed by a sense of futility and self-loathing. This is why it's so important to get started with a belief in yourself and your own ability to succeed again. I frequently remind my clients that it's just a piece of food against them. Food has no life smarts or strategy. It has no I.Q. You have every advantage when you know yourself, your history, and how to approach food situations.

• **At the midpoint.** There's a natural tendency to become less careful when you've started to succeed. Most people on a weight program start to see significant changes in 10 to 30 days. You don't even need to get to the end, to your ideal weight, to see the reward. Your clothes are looser, you're getting compliments, you're happier with yourself, your pain has gone away, and suddenly, you're sliding into old patterns, sabotaging yourself. You may believe that because you've lost a few pounds, you've lost your control problems with certain foods. You may forget that just because the pounds come off, it doesn't mean your history, your taste buds, or your vulnerability to your trigger or problematic foods has changed. Perhaps you're telling yourself that you can handle "just a little." You're feeling a lot less urgency to watch yourself with quantities, to plan ahead, to shop carefully. You become complacent—and complacency is the enemy of thin. Fortunately, there are strategies to save you.

• **At the end.** Success is yours! You've reached your personal best. Every time you look in the mirror, you feel a thrill of pleasure and a sense of pride. The intense satisfaction of achieving your treasured goal convinces you that you'll never go back to your old ways again. Your motivation and commitment are high—for a while. But soon, the honeymoon is over, and you've got to get down to the business of living trim. Maintenance is the most high-risk period of any weight-control effort. Lots of people succeed with dieting— they get an A for dieting every time they stay the course—and then they flunk maintenance. The cause, of course, is usually a lapse in the strategies that are designed not only to carry you through but to help you realize that just because you've lost the weight, you haven't lost the problem.

Many people think about achieving their weight goal in the same way they think about achieving a high school diploma—you get it once and then you can take it for granted for the rest of your life. But food control is an ongoing, dynamic process. And to make the transition from dieting to lifestyle mode requires changing

A Periodic Checkup

For the record, thin doesn't mean qualifying for the cover of *GQ, Shape,* or *Fitness* magazines. By thin, I simply mean your "personal thin." For some, that's the ideal number on the medical charts. For others, personal thin may not be that number—though my wish for each of you is that your weight should be in a healthful range. Yet I realize that if a person is 50 pounds over-weight, and he is motivated or able to lose only 10 to 20 pounds, right now, his life will still be healthier—and this is his personal thin for now.

Throughout this book, when I use the word *fat*, I do not mean it as a judgment, nor as a derogatory term. Fat is simply the word that refers to being medically obese, and I do not attach any judgment to it.

your thinking and staying with the strategies, which will give you the tools for life, to maintain a lifetime of trim.

THE WORK OF HAPPINESS

You probably have always associated diets with deprivation. There is a way around this stumbling block. Put it in the larger context of your life and your most treasured goals—to be happy. It may seem strange in the First Commandment of this book, when there is so much to say about weight control, that I want to talk about the work of happiness. What, you may ask, does that have to do with your losing 10 pounds or 40 or 50 pounds and getting back into your clothes? But from my point of view, happiness and weight loss are very important and intimately connected. The popular mantra of the diet industry is all foods in moderation, but that's a tough trick to pull off when the world we live in isn't given to moderation. It's not enough to want to be trim. You need a plan to get there and stay there. A plan that's livable and doable and that you'll enjoy following—a plan that is about the work of happiness—the happiness that comes from living the vision you have for your own body.

Foods may give you momentary pleasure, but your happiness is the greater reward when you look in the mirror and know you're looking your best, wearing clothes that you've always wanted to wear, feeling fit and glowing with well-being. In our fast-paced culture, the landscape of food is always evolving. In recent decades, the level of food stimuli has increased dramatically. To live in this world and be what I call a selective gourmet—not a compulsive eater—involves strategy.

The role of strategy is to save the foods you love the most and keep them in your life. And it also can let you keep what you care about the most—your appearance, your clothes, your control, and your good health.

As you read the pages of this book and approach your weight-control efforts, stop thinking about dieting. This is what I tell my clients when they first enter my office. It surprises them, until I go on to say that they should *think instead about looking 10 years younger without a face-lift, think in terms of quality of life, self-mastery and growth, fashionable clothes, saving guilt hours at the gym, struggling to make up for yesterday's food excesses. Most of all, I tell them, think about life enhancement—extending and enjoying every day to come of the lives they've been given. I tell them they should think about their highest goals and the work of happiness.*

There is a simple and powerful truth that I will repeat again and again throughout this book: *Being thin may not make you happy, but being fat will make you unhappy.* I can say that on the darkest day of your life, you'll always be happier with yourself if you are living in control with your weight and your food. And I can also say that if you look at the broader picture, *not* living trim and in control will always be harder. Always failing with your weight, never knowing success, always feeling reluctant to face yourself in the mirror or a camera: This is far harder than saying no to a breadbasket, a piece of cake, or any food, or waking up each morning dreading to face the scale, the mirror, or your clothes because of food mistakes.

The goal of the strategies that I present here is not just to change your weight, or change your size, or even to change your behavior—but to change, on the most fundamental level, your thinking. So it's easy to follow all of the other commandments!

There are no good or bad foods.
There are only good or bad histories with a food.

The Second Thin Commandment:
Think Historically,
Not Just Calorically

COMMANDMENT ESSENTIALS

- Think about your food history—how you've behaved with "problem foods" in the past.
- Identify trigger foods, behaviors, situations, and times that lead you to lose control of your eating.
- Stop thinking about simply counting calories, but about how much of your problem food you eat at any one time.
- Realize that even most "healthy" foods aren't healthy if you eat too much of them.

STARTING RIGHT NOW, this book will do something no other diet book has done for you before: It will change your *thinking* about what you eat, and it will change it for the rest of your life.

THE MISSING LINK

Ever since the word "dieting" has been in our language, it has been synonymous with calories and calorie counting. We are taught to think *calorically* about losing weight, and more recently, people are being taught to count the grams of carbohydrates as well. Yet it is this very emphasis on thinking about calories and now carbohydrates that has led millions and millions of people who are successful in so many other things in life to fail utterly at dieting!

Thinking calorically is focusing on the food: what's in the food and how it behaves in your body. Thinking *historically* is all about you: how *you* have behaved with this food over the years of your life and the unique history you have with any food. The problem with the traditional dieting approach is that it is entirely focused on the food: how many calories, how many grams of carbohydrates, how many grams of fat, and so on. Thinking historically shifts the focus to the most critical element for diet success: *you.*

This is the missing link for weight control.

Two people may have a very different history or response to a single 100-calorie cookie. For one person, the cookie may be satisfying—so much so that the person has never abused cookies in his life. For someone else, that one cookie may trigger them to want more and more and even binge on the whole box. Knowing which is true for you may ultimately prove more important to your long-term success at weight control than knowing that the cookie has 100 calories.

When you think historically, you use your whole life experience to evaluate food. Your whole life experience is an immediate predictor of how you will next behave with this food. No weight-control program could possibly discuss every single food you will encounter on your road through life. But by using your own history with food, you have an almost perfect guide.

All you need to do is shift your thinking and ask yourself, "What is my history with this food or this type of food?"

YOUR PERSONAL HISTORY WITH FOOD

Stop and think for a moment what happens whenever you are a new client in a doctor's office: The very first thing you are asked to do is to fill out a detailed questionnaire about your personal medical history. Before any physician attempts a diagnosis, and especially before he prescribes any treatment for you, that physician wants the details of your unique medical history, along with a description of the nature and severity of your symptoms. Only then can you be put on the right path to recovery and lasting health.

As I said in the introduction, *weight control may be the only area of health care where a person's unique food history is totally ignored.* And the consequences have been disastrous. As a professional, it's extremely painful to realize that the dieting field, in its very attempt to help people, has actually led millions and millions—and probably you, the reader—to failure. The need to understand an individual's history with food is the most obvious need in the field of weight control but, tragically, it is the one most overlooked.

The book you have in your hands is the only weight program in the world that teaches you that knowing your own eating history is *first* when it comes to weight control. It comes before learning any calorie tables. For the first time, your eating history is given equal footing with the calories in foods—and this book will explain that in certain situations, respecting your food history is far more important than avoiding excess calories in deciding what to eat.

Every day, weight-control programs and bestselling diet books prescribe one-size-fits-all diets that blatantly violate dieter's food histories. These programs set up dieters for failure, even though they all have only the best intentions. The fact that the vast majority of all people who diet regain the weight they lost is powerful evidence that there is something terribly wrong with the standard approach and recommendations that diet planners and diet books make. If I could make one contribution to the field of weight control, it would be to make the entire field *pay attention to food history* as a central guiding principle.

This is not intended as criticism of my colleagues, who have contributed enormously in the effort to help end obesity. We are all victims of our training, and those who are trained alike, think alike. Fortunately, for the first time in the history of weight control, there really is a dramatic new principle to guide the field: *Think historically, not just calorically.* We can now combine what we know about nutrition, calories, the human body, and human behavior to think in a new way about weight control.

THE KEY TO SUCCESS

When I first started out in the field of weight control, I, like everyone else, thought calorically instead of historically in approaching weight loss. But I was extremely lucky that I soon acquired for a client a very insightful woman named Joan, who runs a very important charity in New York City. Despite all her intelligence, her virtues, and her skills, Joan actually thought of herself as weak-willed and even occasionally "bad" because no matter how many times she disciplined herself to lose weight, her eating and her weight always got out of control.

I worked hard with Joan to make sure she knew exactly the number of calories in every food she was likely to encounter in her busy life. Joan listened carefully and followed my instructions to the letter. She began dropping weight, as she had so many times before. She lost 20 pounds, and her friends began complimenting her on how great she looked. She was delighted to be back into her "best" dress size.

But one night, Joan went to a buffet dinner party where the host was offering a delicious chocolate mousse parfait as dessert along with a tray of little cookies. Quickly calculating that the chocolate mouse had four times as many calories as a couple of cookies, Joan bypassed the mousse and took two cookies instead. That was very good caloric thinking. But *historically,* Joan never had eaten just two cookies in her life! If she ate one, she ate 10. And once Joan ate 10 cookies, she could crave a whole bag of cookies the next day—and the next. Once her cookie cravings started again, Joan couldn't resist them. It was *never* true for Joan that one little cookie was 40 calories. One little cookie was just the first of 5,000 calories a month—with no end in sight!

Had Joan bypassed the cookies and eaten a chocolate mousse parfait for dessert instead, she wouldn't have revived the cycle of cravings and bingeing on cookies that was her unique downfall in dieting, and she would not have regained weight. Joan had no *history* of abusing chocolate mousse in her life. If she ate one serving of mousse, she was satisfied. True, that chocolate mousse would have cost her about 300 calories, but it would have been a one-time splurge. She told me she could have even taken a few tastes and left the remainder. Mousse isn't a food that Joan has a history of eating compulsively, nor is it readily available in her day-to-day environment.

But eating compulsively is exactly what Joan did with cookies. By eating just two cookies, she had reactivated her cravings for more. She started eating them on a regular basis, and soon she was regaining her weight. She left a message at my office saying she wanted to take a break from her appointments.

Most diet books will tell you, and even I believed at the time, that "there are no good foods or bad foods." I discovered that's a dangerous half-truth. The whole truth is: There are no good foods or bad foods. *There are only good and bad histories with a food.*

It was only after months that Joan returned to my office. She gained back even more weight than she had lost. I suggested we take a look at what happened to her in the months since I'd last seen her and what we might learn together. When I carefully retraced with Joan the path that led to her eating spiraling out of control, we both began to suspect that cookies were a trigger that, time and again, propelled Joan into cycles of cravings and bingeing. It was Joan's life-long history with cookies that was primarily responsible for her repeated failures at weight loss. In addition, once she started overeating cookies, she began to let her guard down with other foods as well.

The difference between an occasional dessert for Joan versus compulsively eating cookies offered a powerful clue to her ability to control her weight. Together, we uncovered the key to permanent success at weight control for Joan!

Based on this insight, Joan and I worked out strategies that meant that not only did she not have to give up delicious desserts, but she could even eat satisfying substitutes for cookies that never triggered her cravings. Joan dropped the weight she gained back and has kept it off ever since.

Why It's the Most Essential Strategy

Think historically, not just calorically, is perhaps the most essential strategy of successful weight control. The very instant you begin to think historically, your way of looking at food dramatically changes. You no longer look at the calories in just one cookie, one roll, or one serving of ice cream. Instead, you look at how many cookies, rolls, or scoops of ice cream you *historically* eat, and you can calculate how many calories that one cookie, candy, or scoop of ice cream will ultimately cost you in pounds. I teach my clients to think in "calorie units"—how much they would normally eat based on their history—when they look at a food.

I am frequently interviewed on television and radio about

weight-loss strategies, and I think it's great when talk show hosts are generous enough to share with their audiences their own difficulties with dieting. One male host talked very candidly with me about how hard it was for him to stay in control of his weight given the hectic life he led. When he paused for a commercial break, I watched him finish up a hefty bag of potato chips that his assistant had left near his desk. I leaned over and said to him: "A potato chip has 500 calories." He looked at me as if I were crazy! He showed me the nutrition label on the side of the bag: "A single serving is about 120 calories," he said. I smiled: "Do you always finish the bag?" He confessed he did. So I explained: "If one chip leads you to eat a whole bag of chips that size, then one potato chip is 500 calories— the total number of calories in the bag." Some months later, I was invited back to his program. I complimented him on his weight loss, and before I sat down with him at his desk, he showed me a bag of potato chips—but this time, it was much smaller! "Now one potato chip only has 200 calories." He smiled. "I'll never order the large bag again." And I smiled back and said, "You could be really food smart and buy the *baked* type of potato chips. You'll save even more!"

Diet Plans: Helping or Hurting You?

Of the many clients who came to me only after failing on a low-carb diet such as Atkins, not a single one of them failed because they couldn't live without pasta or eat a lot of meat. They followed the recommended low-carb menus to the letter, but low-carb diets specifically allow the consumption of high-fat cheeses and peanuts. These clients had a long history of abusing just these foods. Some overate the peanuts consistently. Others would lose control with nibbling on the cheeses. Eventually, these clients stopped losing weight, and before long, they were gaining back the weight they had hoped to lose forever.

I had a very motivated client named Carol who came to me frustrated after failing to lose weight on a national weight-control program. The program required that its clients buy the companies' low-calorie meals in advance each week, including all the snacks allowed in the plan. But the problem for Carol turned out to be her long history of compulsively munching finger foods if they were around her house. Once she brought a week's worth of crackers, sugar-free candy, and pretzels into her home, she'd start picking at them. She'd wind up eating a whole week's worth of snacks in the first 2 days alone.

Carol liked the highly organized structure of the weight program, and she wanted to succeed with it. So I suggested to Carol that she skip buying the program's snack foods and instead purchase a single, healthy low-calorie snack each afternoon. (I recommended a yogurt and an apple or a Knight's light popcorn in the small-size bag.) Carol adopted that strategy, and by respecting her unique food history, she began going forward, not backward, on her personal road to being thin, using the meal plans.

GOOD-FOR-YOU FOODS AREN'T ALWAYS GOOD

It's crucial that you realize that very few foods are dietetic or healthy for *you* if *you* have a well-established history of feeding yourself too much of that food. (Although you will find in my diet chapter a list of "free" foods that have made my clients trim.) Newspapers and magazines promote the benefits of eating seven almonds a day, which appears to be a manageable amount of calories in anybody's diet. But I have found that very few people have a history of eating *only* seven almonds and that most people will interpret such well-intentioned advice as a green light to eat handfuls. I've actually never met a man who didn't abuse nuts when eating them by the handful, and I've met many women who share the same problem. The shortsightedness of thinking calorically alone, instead of historically as well, can turn the real cost of seven almonds per day into thousands of excess calories per week!

Studies have shown that people who buy "reduced-fat" snacks end up consuming more calories than those who buy the higher-fat version. Sometimes that's because more sugar has been added to the products, which triggers compulsive eating, but just as often, it's because people who buy foods labeled low-fat or fat-free think it's "safe" to binge on them. I have found the same is true for those who buy the new low-carbohydrate candies, cookies, or ice creams. If they have a history of abusing the high-carb version, they'll also abuse the low-carb versions—even more so!

The mark of smart people is that once they realize that what they have done in the past is not working for them, they change what they are doing. It's a profound shift in your thinking when you begin to consider your personal history with a piece of food *before* you consider the number of calories in the food. When you know your history, you can predict how you will behave with this food or any food in any and all situations. You won't be misled into violating your food history just because a food is low-calorie or "healthy." To shift your thinking, always ask yourself: "What is my history with this food (or this type of food)?" Then—and only then—look at the calories.

FOLLOWING THIS COMMANDMENT

Remember that people like you gain weight because of predictable eating patterns that involve the same foods, the same behaviors, and the same situations.

So how do we discover *your* eating pattern?

When a client first comes to my office, the first thing I do is to explore her food history. I ask her to start by naming any food weaknesses she has. The majority of clients immediately identify either a category of foods, such as sweets, bread products, or salty snacks, or specific foods, such as chocolate or salty chips that trigger them to eat too much of that food. A small minority of clients cite as their eating weakness a particular behavior, nibbling, or eating because they're bored. A handful of my new clients tell me that they repeatedly lose control of their eating when in certain situations, such as cocktail parties and all-you-can-eat buffets.

While each person has her own unique history, all the histories share four common elements that trigger loss of control in eating:

- Trigger foods. People abuse a specific food, whether it is chocolate or bread, or specific types of foods, such as crunchy snacks.
- Trigger behaviors. People repeat a certain specific behavior that leads to overconsumption, such as skipping meals, picking at food with their fingers, or finishing everything on the plate.
- Trigger situations. People repeatedly abuse foods when in certain situations, such as at parties or sports events.
- Trigger times. People abuse food repeatedly at a specific time of the day or week, such as after dinner or while relaxing on Sunday afternoons. Ninety percent of my clients report little problems with food until the mid-to-late afternoon (typically starting around 3 or 4 P.M.) on into the evening.

I think of an individual's unique pattern of eating as her "eating print." Just like you have your own unique fingerprint, you have your own unique eating print too. Your eating print is a *dynamic* pattern of foods, behaviors, and situations that trigger you to lose control of your eating. It is a repetitive pattern that forms a predictable mosaic of your own personal food weaknesses and eating behaviors. Recognizing your own eating print is one of the single most powerful tools you can use to gain control of your weight.

In psychology, there is an axiom that if you do what you have always done, you will get the result you have always gotten. You can't do what you have always done and expect to get a different result. That's why knowing your eating print and learning the new strategies in this book can end your cycle of weight gain forever. You can enjoy a wide variety of delicious foods without wearing them—but only if you know your own history!

WHAT ARE YOUR TRIGGER FOODS?

Identifying a trigger food is as simple as it looks. Ask yourself: "Is this food a weakness of mine? Do I eat one piece (or a single serving) of this food—or 10?" What are the foods that give you the greatest cravings that have also contributed to your greatest weight problems? Your mouth may water at the thought of your sister-in-law's homemade mushroom barley soup, but soup isn't making you gain weight. Some of you already know your trigger foods under another name: "comfort foods." In a recent issue of *More* magazine, a reader wrote in: "Comfort foods for me are mashed potatoes, cookies, and chocolates. But I've finally learned to eat foods that make me feel good *afterward:* fruits, vegetables, fiber, and low-fat dairy." That is a woman who knows her food history and is using smart strategies to deal with it!

The F-Q Principle

One of the hallmarks of a trigger food is that at the beginning of a diet, you usually give it up, out of an intuitive feeling that it will impede your weight control. But once you've lost an amount of weight that pleases you, you feel it's "safe" to go back to it. At first, you are very focused on not abusing that food. You'll only eat one cookie or a single breadstick from the breadbasket and walk away from the rest. But it's the beginning of the road backward, although you seldom realize it. If you're thinking calorically, the logic of going back to your old ways proves almost irresistible in the coming days: You had a cookie or a few nibbles from the breadbasket and didn't put on any weight, so why not do it again? And again? I call it the F-Q Principle because once the *frequency* starts to increase, invariably the *quantity* will increase as well, until it reaches the amount it was before. And you will gain back the amount of weight you lost before! Thinking calorically, there is nothing wrong with eating one cookie or starting to pick on a few breadsticks from the breadbasket in front of you. Yet this behavior is a bridge back to a pattern of behavior that may be marked by a long history of overeating, proving once again that history comes before calories!

No More Trigger Foods—Forever?

Once you identify your trigger foods and recognize the role that they are playing in your weight gain, *must* you give them up? Most likely not. Giving up your trigger foods forever is just *one* smart strategy in weight control. Many of my clients use a variety of smart strategies (you will learn many of them in the section on "boxing in" a food on page 83) that either enable them to keep those foods in their life or switch to substitute foods that they find equally pleasurable.

TRIGGER BEHAVIORS

New clients sometimes tell me they don't have any food weaknesses at all: They overeat all foods, they say, and they believe that's why they are overweight. What they really mean is that they *finish* all foods. "Finishing" is a behavior that triggers overconsumption, just like picking at food with your fingers is another kind of behavior that triggers overconsumption. Once you know you have a history of being a "finisher," you can learn strategies to avoid being served fattening foods in a restaurant, so that whatever you finish isn't going to make you heavy. Likewise, once you know you have a history of overconsuming finger foods, even a strategy as simple as always eating your pizza with a knife and fork can stop you from gaining weight. Or when you're at a party, carry a glass of appetite-quenching tomato juice in one hand and a crunchy crudité in the other. For some people, *the essence of weight control is simply finger control.*

Other kinds of behaviors that lead people to overeat are skipping meals, going food shopping after work, waiting so long to eat that you arrive at a restaurant so starved that you demolish the breadbasket, or overeating at a buffet or family-style restaurant. If you have a history of routinely engaging in these types of behaviors, you will find that the Fourth Thin Commandment, Structure Gives Control, is filled with strategies that address precisely these issues (see page 52).

TRIGGER TIMES AND SITUATIONS

One of the most predictable and fascinating things about dieters is that if they gain back the weight they lost, they will not only do it with the same foods and the same behaviors, they will do it in the *same places* and at the *same times* that they gained that weight the first time around. Buffets, salad bars, and all-you-can-eat restaurants trigger overconsumption for many people. It can also be that a certain day of the week, like having long hours of free time on a weekend afternoon, triggers some people to overeat. Many of my clients report that they have no problems with food until the hours between 4 o'clock and 5 o'clock every afternoon—those are the times that they fall prey to the foods and eating behaviors that cause them to gain weight.

To help raise your level of awareness, I've ranked the top three problem-eating times in order of frequency:

1. Later afternoon

2. Evenings—while waiting for dinner

3. Weekend afternoons at home

Very few people tend to overeat in the morning or the early part of the day.

THE PREDICTABILITY OF
YOUR EATING BEHAVIOR

If you see that never in your entire lifetime have you been able to eat just seven nuts, or skip breakfast without gorging later, nor can

How Does This Commandment Make You a Weight-Control Winner?

1. It predicts your behavior in advance with any food you have eaten in your life.
2. It predicts the time of the day when you are most likely to be vulnerable to overeating.
3. It predicts the types of situations that are most associated with losses of control.
4. It helps you evaluate food in a new way—not just in terms of counting calories and carbohydrates, but in terms of how any food affects your behavior, appetite, control, and success at dieting.
5. It helps you set up boundaries that come out of your own unique life history and break through the feelings of deprivation that haunt your own life.
6. It shifts your thinking from being "good" or "bad" to thinking in terms of "what works or doesn't work for me."

you stay away from chips on a weekend, you can predict with certainty that you will gain weight by continuing down that path. Or you can take control of your life by learning the strategies that will change your history and create a happier future for yourself.

Predictability is the highest goal of all science. Knowing your own history hands you the key to the *most* scientific approach you will ever find to losing weight. When you can predict in advance your responses to food based on your history and use strategy accordingly, you stop being a victim who marches blindly through the world of food, tripping over the same potholes again and again.

When you understand your own food history, you finally understand that it's not the whole world of food against you. Nor is the whole world of dieting against you. When you think in terms of your own unique food history *first,* you see that the problem may never have been with you at all, but with the food itself.

Each person is a living textbook of one. There is tremendous biological variability in our species, so what may be completely unappealing to someone else may drive you into an eating frenzy.

The Third Thin Commandment:
The Problem May Be in the Food, Not in You

COMMANDMENT ESSENTIALS

- Kill appetite cravings with a sweet protein shake when fruit won't do the trick.
- Don't skip meals or go too long without eating.
- Eat a protein or a protein with high fiber for breakfast.
- Substitute pickles or spicy V-8 juice when tempted to indulge in sweets.
- Never try to correct for overeating by skipping meals the following day.
- Be aware of SAD cold-weather eating.
- Keep your home a "junk food–free" zone.

THE FOLLOWING SCENARIO IS as predictable as a Hollywood action movie. Call it *Diet Terminator.* You commit yourself to losing weight. You have all the best intentions of sticking with a diet and actually do so for a while. Until . . . a tray of cookies shoots you a tempting glance. Or you inhale the riveting aroma of a pizza bubbling in a brick oven, or perhaps you'll just have a few nuts from that bowl of cashews. The next thing you know, you're sitting in a bloated stupor, wondering how a tiny bite of food led to eating so much more than you ever intended. You call yourself weak and undisciplined and think that you have no willpower. You might even suspect that you have an eating disorder.

You may be dead wrong. A whole new field of scientific research is emerging that may explain why you have failed so often in your dieting. This research is exploring how the foods you eat today may change the chemistry of your brain in such a way as to increase your appetite and cravings for these and other foods—even without you being aware that this process is taking place.

Just as the first chapter discussed changing your thinking, so this chapter will address your physical makeup and its influence on your food choices and teach you how to be a winner at weight control. You'll learn about the physiological basis of appetite, why you may be having recurring problems controlling certain foods, and how to make your body work *for* you, not against you. Using this knowledge, you'll be able to reduce or even eliminate your cravings for certain foods and, for the first time, have the power to take control of foods that have sabotaged your weight loss again and again.

These new studies may even change your own perception of yourself as a person lacking willpower, as someone who has never succeeded on a diet because you lacked backbone.

Thanks to the latest scientific research, we've learned that while *weight control is primarily about balancing calories in and calories out, appetite and craving control is about the types of foods you eat and how they interact with your body's genetic and chemical hardwiring. In short, the problem may be in the food, not in you.*

In fact, what may surprise you is that your eating behavior and the very foods you choose for breakfast, lunch, and dinner today may be influenced by the interaction of the food with your genetics and neurochemistry. This process is going on without your knowing it, which is why you may overconsume these foods without intending to. (Remember those promises to yourself: "I'll have just one"?) It may also explain why you keep regaining the same weight with the same foods, despite the best of intentions.

Now, as science is revealing that the problem may be in the food, not in you, the good news is that even if you have genetic sensitivities to certain foods, all you need are the right strategies to manage them. And for those of you who prefer to get a certain food out of your life completely, I'll provide the powerful tools to not only make it possible, but easy.

So if you have an uncontrollable craving for a particular food that unleashes a furious eating bender, you'll be relieved to discover that this urge doesn't prove that you are a spineless mess with a weak character. Or that you can't succeed at weight control. All it proves is that you are human—and you need strategy.

DOES OUR DNA RULE OUR APPETITES?

Genes exert a tremendous influence over both our biology—they give us such things as red hair and blue eyes—and our behavior. *But up to now, we've never realized genes' influence over our eating habits, our appetites, and the type of diet we should follow—and even whether or not we'll succeed on that diet.*

Your genes may send powerful, unconscious messages that impel you to, say, make a beeline for the pastry cart or to accumulate more than a few extra pounds of fat. While these urges can cause us grief, they have a sound basis in evolution. As Terry Burnham and Jay Phelan write in their book *Mean Genes,* "Our ancestors lived off the land by hunting animals and gathering plants . . . Just staying alive required lots of energy—energy that could be found only in food . . ." What kept our ancestors going in a tough, physically demanding world? Hunger. Our ancestors needed to stay hungry day and night; their only goal was storing enough food to keep them alive during the inevitable lean times. And they sought not just any kind of food, but calorically dense, fatty foods. But while this kind of gluttony was necessary for survival in the Neolithic African bush, in our ultra-convenient, sedentary society of plenty, it only leads to expanding waistlines.

Scientists have clearly established that for many of us, our genes play a large role in controlling our weight, as confirmed by the following discoveries:

- Hereditary factors can impact our appetites.
- Genes may regulate how efficiently we convert food into energy, which can affect our weight.
- In 2002, scientists discovered a gene, HOB1, that they promptly labeled the "fat gene." They've also identified from

eight to 30 other genes that may contribute to obesity by in-
hibiting the body's metabolism.
- Researchers at the Monell Chemical Senses Center are
working on discovering a "sweet tooth" gene that would locate a person's vulnerability to sweet cravings.

JUMP-START YOUR APPETITE

Hormones are complex molecules produced by the endocrine
glands that manage many bodily functions and processes. One of
the most important hormones for appetite is insulin, the "hunger
hormone," which the body uses to process glucose (sugar) and me-
diate our cravings for fat and carbohydrates. The level of insulin also
influences the storage of calories as fat and even the degree to which
we may be able to lose weight on a particular diet.

When blood glucose rises, your pancreas produces insulin,
which converts the excess glucose to glycogen (glucose stored in
the liver) or fat. When your blood glucose dips too low, and you
don't replenish it by eating, your body siphons glycogen. Normally,
this process is neatly balanced, and insulin and other hormones help
you maintain a stable body weight.

However, your diet can shatter this equilibrium. If you consume large amounts of refined simple carbohydrates, *and* you're significantly overweight (especially with abdominal fat), you can cause
the pancreas to become a superproductive insulin factory, creating
the condition known as "insulin resistance."

A person with insulin resistance has to produce more insulin to
reduce his blood glucose to normal levels, according to Walter Futterweit, M.D., clinical professor of medicine and for many years
chief of the Endocrine Clinics at the Mt. Sinai School of Medicine
in New York City, and one of America's leading endocrinologists.
The increasing amounts of insulin lead to hyperinsulinism—too
much of it in the body. All that insulin can increase your appetite
and lead to fatigue, lack of concentration, shakiness, sweats, and an
excessive lowering of blood sugar called reactive hypoglycemia. At
this point, you may try to get relief by taking in more and more
simple carbohydrates, which only causes more insulin production in
a damaging cycle. It's important to note that even if you are not in-

sulin resistant, but you go too long without eating, you can create a state of induced reactive hypoglycemia with the same cravings and symptoms.

In working with thousands of clients, it has been my observation that a large number of them have had insulin cravings for carbohydrates, and giving them a diet that includes such foods as cookies, pasta, bagels, and sugary breakfast cereals may actually increase their cravings for more and lead to a heightened appetite throughout the day.

A study conducted by Peter Havel of the University of California and Michael Schwartz of the University of Washington also revealed that *over time,* a diet high in fat and fructose (a sugar very frequently found in healthy products such as many bran muffins and baked goods) may affect insulin levels and increase appetite. *The food itself is actually increasing the person's cravings, appetite, and hunger level.* What's worse, Schwartz says, is that the brain loses its ability to respond to insulin as a person gets fatter and/or when fat is more than 30 percent of the person's diet. Under these conditions, tissues also may become insensitive to insulin, and carbohydrate cravings are intensified.

In June 2004, a study by researchers at the Monell Center in Philadelphia also suggested that overconsumption of fructose seems to alter appetite-regulating hormones in a way that stimulates overeating.

People in the study who ate a meal followed by a drink containing the same amount of fructose as that found in two cans of soda showed relatively low levels of insulin and leptin (another hormone that signals to people that they are full), and higher levels of ghrelin, a hormone that stimulates eating.

According to Sarah Leibowitz, Ph.D., a professor at the Rockefeller University laboratory of behavioral neuroscience in New York City and one of the preeminent researchers of the physiological basis of eating behavior and weight, hormones also have been known to increase appetite and craving for sweets or meat in women with premenstrual syndrome. The hormones are acting under the evolutionary pressure of genes; it's nature's way of telling a woman that she needs extra fat calories if she wants to produce a child.

Finally, stress—whether physical or psychological—also can

Carb Cravings and Why You Can't Lose Weight

Millions of women may not be aware that they have a condition that is making it difficult for them to lose weight and fueling cravings for carbohydrates, especially sweets.

Polycystic ovary syndrome (PCOS) is a serious condition that affects 5 to 9 percent of the women of reproductive age; half of these women are overweight.

Women with PCOS suffer irregular menstrual cycles during adolescence; their symptoms may also include acne and other skin conditions, irregular hair growth, or thinning hair.

From 30 to 40 percent of obese patients with PCOS, at the time they're first seen by a physician, already have an abnormally high tolerance for sugar and an increased frequency of type 2 diabetes, says Dr. Walter Futterweit, one of the world's premiere authorities on PCOS, whose groundbreaking studies have helped identify the mechanisms of PCOS.

Both high insulin levels and insulin resistance are very common in this syndrome, which explains why many women with PCOS have increased cravings for sweets. And after they eat cookies, candies, sweet juices, or other carbohydrates such as pasta, they often develop other symptoms such as sleepiness, lack of concentration, and occasional shakiness and sweatiness. In addition, diets with even a limited amount of these foods may make it extremely difficult for them to lose weight—even though they may be restricting calories. If you suspect that you have this condition, you should consult your physician. (You can also find more information from the Polycystic Ovarian Syndrome Association at 877-775-PCOS or at www.pcosupport.org.)

Women with PCOS have trouble losing weight while their diet contains high or even medium amounts of carbohydrates. Dr. Futterweit advises women with PCOS to go on a low-carbohydrate diet and eat small meals throughout the day, always including some protein when they eat carbohydrates. An eating plan such as one given in this book, based on low-fat protein, nonstarchy vegetables, healthy monounsaturated oil found in seafood and fish, poultry, eggs, and low-fat dairy, plus limited amounts of fruit, would be ideal for women with this condition. If you switch to this way of eating, you should find a decrease in your craving for carbohydrates and an increase in your weight loss.

wreak havoc with weight control by releasing the so-called stress hormones—adrenaline, corticotrophin-releasing hormone (CRH), and cortisol—to meet what the body perceives as an emergency. High amounts of cortisol may cause deposits of fat around the midsection. Stress also depletes your body's glycogen fuel reserves. And the longer and more intense the stress, the lower your blood sugar will dip, which often leads to carbohydrate cravings. *Yes, your stress may make you hungry and cause you to store more fat.*

And, of course, one of our favorite ways to relieve stress is by reaching for the nearest candy bar or cookie, which leads to higher insulin levels and carb cravings in what can be a destructive loop of perpetual craving and eating.

So as you can see, the hormones in your blood and the chemicals in your brain perform a delicate balancing act that requires smart food strategies to avoid trouble. And you'll learn some very creative strategies to master stress and lose weight comfortably in the Fifth Commandment, Separate Mood from Food (see page 68).

CAN YOU BE ADDICTED TO A LAYER CAKE?

Dopamine is a neurotransmitter—a molecule that sends messages from one neuron in the brain to another—produced by an enzymatic pathway in the brain. It's been called the "feel-good molecule." It creates pleasurable sensations in your brain every time you have sex, hear your favorite music, dig into an ice cream sundae, or (unfortunately) use cocaine. Scientists have isolated it as a key to understanding drug and alcohol addiction.

While drugs such as alcohol, cocaine, and opiates seem to boost the release of dopamine and other neurochemicals involved in the change in thought and behavior that characterize addictive states, recent findings suggest that these same neurochemicals may be involved even when we form dependencies on such things as coffee, cake, or gambling. And scientists such as Harvard psychiatry professor Hans Breiter have discovered through magnetic resonance imaging that the same brain centers that are activated during the ecstasy of drug use also do so in compulsive gamblers on a "high."

This suggests the conclusion that not only drug use but any recurring activity that triggers dopamine release, such as eating certain foods, can reshape the brain in important ways—ways that compel you to keep repeating that action and that make "Just saying no" much more difficult. Scientists call this neuroadaptation, and it could at least partially explain why you can't stop yourself from wolfing down those chocolate-covered raisins. (This is not to say that dopamine is the only chemical involved in the thought processes of drug abusers or addictive-like behaviors.)

While I'm careful not to overuse the term "addiction," a leading expert has pointed out, "if you look at all addictions from tobacco to heroin, there's only one clear statement that applies to all of them: uncontrolled use despite negative consequences." Our present epidemic of obesity and compulsive eating may share some remarkable similarities of behavior and neurobiology with that observation.

It's important to realize when we speak about an addictive or addictive-like relationship with a substance or a food that the research holds out the hope that this relationship can be reversed through learning.

Journalist Madeleine Nash, in a very revealing article on addictive behavior in *Time* magazine, came to an important insight after reviewing the studies and various modalities of treatment: "One of the most hopeful messages coming out of current research is that the biochemical abnormalities associated with addiction can be reversed through learning. For that reason, all sorts of psychological interventions, ranging from psychotherapy to 12-Step programming, can and do help. Cognitive therapy, which seeks to supply people with coping skills—exercising after work instead of going to a bar—appears to hold particular promise. After just 10 weeks of therapy, before-and-after PET-scans [positive emission tomography] of the brain suggest that some patients suffering from obsessive-compulsive disorders manage to resculpt not only their behavior but also activity patterns in their brain." Having developed strategies for thousands of compulsive eaters that helped them to lose the cravings and the interest in foods they had been out of control with for decades, I can only say, "Amen!"

Perhaps most significant in this analysis is that teaching people coping skills not only changes their behavior but may change the brain activity that underlies it. That's why strategy is so critical in managing certain types of foods.

In the end, you should listen to your body when it comes to food. Just because your symptoms may not meet someone's textbook definition of addiction doesn't mean they don't exist. And as we shall see now, there is another factor that may impel you to act like an addict by craving more and more carbohydrates or fueling your appetite and a cycle of compulsive overeating.

NEUROPEPTIDE Y: THE MISSING LINK IN CRAVING CONTROL?

Up to now, we've been talking about genetics and environmental and neurochemical factors and their instinctive influence on your eating. However, *to a large degree, your response to food is primarily in your own hands*. A classic example of how your behavior influences the control of appetite and the success of your diet is the case of neuropeptide Y.

Have you ever noticed that if you've gone a number of hours without eating, skipped meals, or just eaten too little, by a certain part of the day, usually the late afternoon, your appetite starts to rev up? Well, so does almost everybody else's. In a recent survey reported in *Shape* magazine, 98 percent of participants in a weight-control program said they tend to overeat at the same time each day.

Why is this? Dr. Sarah Leibowitz's studies suggest that this clockwork craving may be caused by surging levels of a protein known as neuropeptide Y, which may contribute to "a stimulatory effect on food intake, particularly carbohydrate ingestion."

While Dr. Leibowitz's groundbreaking research focuses on animals, C. Wayne Calloway, M.D., an endocrinologist at George Washington University in Washington, D.C., is a clinician working with weight-control patients. He explained to *Allure* magazine, "If the body has been deprived of sufficient calories during the day, the levels of metabolic regulator neuropeptide Y will rise once one starts eating. This leads to greater cravings for food, especially carbohydrates . . . At that point, it's hard to resist the body's chemical signals to consume. You turn into an eating automaton, without being aware of it. If you think you're an intelligent, responsible person, it's spooky how little control you have over this."

Neuropeptide Y is so powerful that it imprints whatever you

eat on an empty stomach on your brain's craving control center. And those foods—especially simple carbs such as sweets, refined flour products, and baked goods—deactivate your appetite-control mechanism and may ignite increased cravings for more and more, even though you intend to "have just a little."

It's very critical to understand the interaction of all these processes, which combine to make so many people feel like they lack willpower to fight their seemingly insatiable appetite. When the truth is that if you've gone beyond a few hours without eating, then having a cookie, that cookie, instead of satisfying you, becomes a turbocharged appetite stimulant causing you to overeat. This can be true even if you've never craved cookies before, a fact proven by a 1990 study at University College, London, in which subjects who were indifferent to chocolate but ate it on an empty stomach ended up craving it.

Can a Craving Be Unlearned?

The same British researchers who discovered that people who didn't particularly care for chocolate developed cravings for it when they ate it on an empty stomach may also have found a way to "unlearn" a craving. Chocolate junkies who ate half a bar immediately after lunch and half a bar immediately after dinner for 2 weeks lost their craving for chocolate. The key to losing the craving appears to rest in (1) eating it when you're not hungry and the stomach is full (this is critical), and (2) "flooding yourself" with the taste of the food by having it repeatedly (i.e., twice a day) for 2 weeks. Apparently, no matter how much you like a food or how much it has retarded your progress at weight control, you may be able to extinguish your cravings for it. You can use this same technique to eliminate or reduce cravings for foods that have held back your progress at weight control. But beware the reverse can also be true; if you eat it on an empty stomach or in place of a meal, you can increase your cravings!

Food Memories and the "Proust Factor"

In Marcel Proust's classic, *In Search of Lost Time,* the autobiographical protagonist, Marcel, bites into a tea cookie called a madeleine, which generates a memory of when he first sampled the cookie as a child. From this reminiscence, a tidal wave of other memories and associations washes over him (enough to fill seven volumes!).

Proust's "appetite memory" led to the creation of a literary masterpiece. But this kind of powerful recollection can also create cravings for certain foods. It could be years since you tasted that special cookie, but one bite would bring back the longing for its sugary chewiness. This thought is called an "emotional memory."

Along with these memories, cravings can be triggered by the visual stimulus of food and its aroma, which produce neurochemical changes in the brain that ignite its appetite craving center. Numerous studies show that the more foods you see and keep around your home, the more you eat and the more frequently you eat—even if you're not hungry. And let's face it, in our culture, food is everywhere—all around your house, in 24-hour restaurants and supermarkets, and buffets in conference rooms and meetings. Kelly Brownell, a professor of psychology at Yale, has wisely described this as a "toxic food environment"—and your own home may be the most toxic.

Whether it's genes or behavior, nature or nurture, eating behavior for many of us habituates very quickly. I call it the power of "just one bite." For example, many of my clients who eat in restaurants make a decision not to touch the breadbasket and go many weeks, months, or even years abstaining. The breadbasket stops being a major source of temptation, and they may even stop being aware of it. Then they're tempted one evening by the aroma of a freshly baked roll in a fine restaurant. One leads to two, and soon enough, they've gone back to ransacking the breadbasket. First, they eat it out of preference; then they eat it out of habit.

For Proust, an emotional memory was a bridge back to the past of his idealized childhood, but for you, it could be a bridge back to a time or place when you abused foods—a past you'd rather not revisit.

TASTE BUDS: A CRITICAL KEY TO APPETITE CONTROL

There is yet another reason why so many of my clients may be able to have "just one" cookie, then stop eating, while a second person can go from one cookie to 10 in no time flat. It has to do with the number of taste buds, the groups of cells on our tongue that distinguish between sweet and bitter, salty and creamy. So often my clients have asked me why they don't have the willpower of their spouse to have just one cookie. I look at them and smile and say, "He may not have more willpower than you, but he may have more taste buds on his tongue."

Linda Bartoshuk, a professor of the Yale University School of Medicine, has conducted years of pioneering research on taste buds that I believe will have strong implications for weight control. She has discovered that some people may have a few hundred taste buds on their tongue, while others have tens of thousands. The former group, called "nontasters," has a high tolerance for and often desire fatty, salty, and bitter foods, which cause them to indulge in them more frequently.

On the other hand, the "supertasters" have highly sensitive palates. Food "floods" over them; sweet tastes a lot sweeter and fat a lot fatter. They're easily repulsed by bitter flavors. In the middle are "medium tasters."

The supertasters are perfectly sated by one cookie. But by the time the nontasters reach their point of satiety, they've taken in so much sugar, flour, and/or fat that it's affecting their neurochemistry and setting in motion overconsumption or binge eating.

Taste bud differential may also explain why some people can't have "just one" potato chip for "crunch"—and why salt may serve

Test Your Taste Buds

There are two simple ways for you to determine what kind of taster you are. (1) Put some saccharine on the tip of your tongue. If you taste only sweetness, you are probably a nontaster. But if you taste sweetness and bitterness, you're most likely a medium taster. If the saccharine tastes extremely bitter, you're a supertaster. (2) Put some blue food coloring on the tip of your tongue. If you're a supertaster, your tongue will look covered in pink dots, called fungiform papillae. If you're a medium taster, you'll see half white dots and half pink dots. If your tongue looks more polka-dotted, with many fewer pink dots, you're probably a nontaster.

as a major appetite trigger. You see, if the potato chip was soggy, they would have no trouble stopping at one. (To find out what kind of taster you are, see the box, "Test Your Taste Buds" on page 44.)

This research is only in its infancy, and among other things, we're learning that gender and race seem to have an effect on the number of taste buds you have. Thirty-five percent of women are more likely to be supertasters, as opposed to only 15 percent of men. And more Asians than Caucasians are supertasters, which means they often find sugary foods cloying and prefer less sweet desserts. That's why none of my clients has ever gone to a Japanese or Chinese restaurant in a desperate search for a dessert!

However, the critical point is that an inborn, genetic predisposition influences how powerfully we respond to the taste and texture of food. What is sickeningly sweet to one person may prove to be the ultimate treat to another. A second crucial point is made by Valerie Duffy, Ph.D., an assistant professor of dietetics at the University of Connecticut: "People tend to look at someone who's overweight and say, 'He has no willpower' or 'Why can't she just walk away from food?' When the truth is that it just may be easier for some people to turn down certain foods because of their taste bud structure." As Dr. Duffy implies, *This is not about willpower,* as illustrated by the following anecdote:

The work of Drs. Bartoshuk, Duffy, and other taste bud researchers suggests that (1) people may live "in different worlds of taste"; (2) this biological variability influences how much you will typically eat of a certain food; i.e., whether you can consume it moderately or abuse it; (3) why some people are "finishers" of certain foods—they'll always feel compelled to finish a dessert while others are satisfied with a taste; and most important, (4) your taste preferences may influence what types of food you buy in the supermarket or order in a restaurant and how much you weigh.

Taste bud research also may help us understand that the dynamics of compulsive eating for many may be more accurately explained in terms of physiology rather than psychopathology. These studies, along with the neuropeptide Y phenomenon, clearly lend credence to one of the favorite adages I have imparted to my clients—"You don't have to be crazy to be crazy about a cookie!"

A genetic sensitivity to sugar or salt plus very few taste buds, which typically leads to overconsuming, can easily become a dangerous mix. Since nontasters may need to consume a large quantity of sugary or salty foods to feel satisfied, they trigger a tremendous amount of insulin, the hunger hormone. So instead of eating just one or two cookies, they find themselves finishing the whole box.

The good news is that with strategy, you'll soon *learn to handle your physiology and still keep your favorite foods in your life—and remain your favorite size!*

HOW WILL THIS COMMANDMENT HELP YOU?

What can we learn from the scientific research discussed in this chapter to increase success at weight control and to make it easy? By understanding how the timing of your eating and the types of foods you eat affect your appetite, you have the knowledge to change your attitude and then your behavior. Here's what this commandment provides:

⬧ It relieves guilt by helping you understand that any binges or compulsive overeating may not be due to personal weakness but

If You Sleep Too Little, You Could Eat Too Much

Sometimes my clients tell me they've been hungry all week. In helping them figure out the reason for their hunger, I ask them if they've been sleeping properly. They often look surprised at this question—but they shouldn't be. Sleep deprivation is known to jump-start your appetite, particularly carbohydrate cravings. Studies have demonstrated that depriving both lab animals and humans of sleep increased both their appetites and food consumption. One study of college students found that getting only 2½ hours of sleep for 3 nights in a row and interrupting their sleep on 3 other nights greatly increased their appetite. Another study of young men who were deprived of REM sleep demonstrated a marked increase in appetite.

may instead be a reflection of powerful, complex biochemical forces and how they interact with certain foods you select—and at what time of the day and under what conditions you eat them.

• It helps you realize that all your previous failures at weight control may have had very little to do with a lack of willpower, but instead a lack of strategy to deal with your genetic sensitivity.

• It points the way to possible solutions—such as food shopping and dining strategies that help you control salty or sweet foods or foods with creamy and/or crunchy textures—if you think you're bingeing or you think you have an eating disorder.

• It describes the types of foods that won't trigger overconsumption and warns you of the ones that will.

• It explains why, if you haven't eaten for several hours, and you then eat simple carbohydrates such as low-fiber crackers, candies, cookies, and chips, you may find yourself getting increasingly hungry and overconsuming for the next few hours.

• It helps to explain why, if you can't stop to eat during the day (or if you eat too little), you may find you can't stop eating at night.

• It helps you understand which foods you're hypersensitive to and why your family or friends can have a taste of this food, but if *you* start, you feel a compulsive need for more and more.

• It helps you understand that you may live in a different world of taste and that you should adjust your food choices to succeed in that world.

• It reveals research suggesting that breakfasts made of simple carbs such as instant oats, low-fiber sugary breakfast cereals, or the American favorite, bagels, may actually trigger appetite and lead to increased consumption for the entire day.

• It changes our notion of what makes a good snack for weight and appetite control. Most weight programs allow you a snack in between meals. Make certain this snack is one that does not trigger appetite and cravings.

• It suggests that diets recommended by certain weight-control programs, which ignore your food history and don't take into account your genetic sensitivity to certain foods or snacks or provide any strategies to deal with them, may actually be causing you to have cravings, lose control, and fail at the very diet they are trying to help you follow.

In subsequent chapters, I'll present a wide range of successful strategies to help you lose weight and keep it off. However, if you abandon these strategies and go head to head with your physiology, the likelihood that you'll succeed is very small.

Tips for Ending Your Cravings

One of the most powerful observations we can draw from the neuropeptide Y and British craving research is that we have the power to either end or diminish our cravings or to fuel them to an unmanageable level, often unknowingly. A lot of the people who feel that they're doomed to fail because of their cravings for high-caloric foods or foods they continually abuse can now use the following strategies to end the cravings.

- Don't skip meals or go too long without eating.
- Start your day with a breakfast that doesn't trigger hunger or increased carbohydrate cravings later on.
- Eat a protein or a protein with high fiber for breakfast (which is the best breakfast for many people), such as yogurt with fresh fruit sprinkled with a few tablespoons of high-fiber cereal such as All-Bran. Alternately, try an omelet (or egg-white/egg substitute omelet) with fresh vegetables and/or low-fat cheese, or try my recommended GG Scandinavian Bran Crispbread (the only high-fiber cracker I've ever found that has a sum total of zero net carbs and a mere 16 calories)—literally a crunchy carb without carbs—with Laughing Cow Light cheese wedges melted over it.
- If you like to eat cereal for breakfast, I've found that a high-fiber cereal with protein, such as All-Bran or Fiber One with fat-free milk, doesn't stimulate appetite later in the day for most people. Be careful to measure out a single serving. (Most people typically pour an indiscriminate amount into their breakfast bowl that may be three or four times the calories on the box plus the extra milk calories.)
- Make protein or a protein combined with a high-fiber food your snack of choice for that late-afternoon or early evening period. (See Part 2, starting on page 173, for recommendations.)
- Don't be tricked by many so-called health-food snacks such as cereal or granola bars, which often have single-digit grams of fiber and double-digit grams of sugar or fructose.

• Try a heavy, liquid sweet, such as a sweet protein shake, to kill appetite and cravings safely when fruit is unsatisfying or actually increases cravings/appetites in the later afternoon (when neuropeptide Y is rising).

• Be aware of SAD cold-weather eating. *Those suffering from SAD who experience increased appetite cravings or cravings for carbohydrates can still find success at weight control during the winter months with healthy carbohydrates that are sweet such as baked sweet potatoes, the previously suggested sweetened bran crackers, or high-fiber waffles.* Whether or not you suffer from SAD, the winter months may bring a shift in food preferences toward hot and heavy meals.

• Detoxify your home food environment. This starts at your supermarket and ends in your refrigerator and cabinets. Strive to set up an eating and living environment conducive to healthful living.

• Limit post-exercise snacks or meals to foods high in protein and/or fiber or a high-fiber low-carbohydrate variety.

• Never try to correct an overeating/bingeing error by skipping meals or eating miniscule amounts of food the next day. Doing so will only fuel further overconsumption by the end of the day. Instead, eat full meals that offer large volume but low calories such as seafood and low-fat omelets. A less-satisfactory alternative would be low-fat meats such as turkey, pork, or reduced-fat chicken cutlets.

• Never go hungry to restaurants or events such as meetings or conferences where food is available. That's because the first thing you may be confronted with is a breadbasket, baked goods, or candy, which will trigger the neuropeptide Y storm and, later, hunger and cravings.

• Realize that seeing and smelling foods you love—or even reading about them—can trip your appetite alarm, even when you're not hungry.

• Be aware that as a nontaster (which means that you need large amounts of sweets and/or salt to fill you up), eating a small amount may be very difficult for you physiologically. *Correct for this by buying a single-size serving at the supermarket, or order it in a controlled setting such as a restaurant, where you'll be given a single serving.*

Once again, in evaluating all of these strategies, use your own food history as the ultimate litmus test of how your body will respond to the food in question and the need for control strategies.

The taste bud and neuropeptide Y research can also be used in reverse, to encourage consumption of healthy foods you do not like. Here's what to do to help dupe your tongue into savoring foods that ordinarily repel it:

- Add a small amount of salt or spice when cooking pungent vegetables such as cauliflower and brussels sprouts, or blanch them in salt for a couple of minutes before you eat them. Salt blocks bitterness. To avoid excess salt, try a splash of balsamic vinegar, lemon juice, or low-sodium soy sauce.
- Top those hard-to-swallow veggies with some sautéed bread crumbs or a little crumbly light/fat-free cheese. (You can even find fat-free feta and low-fat goat cheese in many supermarkets.)
- Add 2 tablespoons of the above kinds of cheese or the same amount of raisins to your salad.
- Sprinkle a pinch of sugar or a low-glycemic sweetener such as stevia or one of the sugar-free maple syrups such as Walden Farms Calorie-Free on your grapefruit or other tart fruits. This strategy will also work for a cup of plain yogurt, so you can avoid the high sugar of many low-fat/fat-free yogurts.

GENES IMPEL; THEY DON'T COMPEL

One of the greatest rewards and passions of my work has not only been to lift the pain of pounds of fat and a lifelong history of failure in thousands of individuals, but most of all to end years of guilt and self-blame and rid people of the notion that they have a psychopathology, eating disorder, or lack the strength of willpower. When I explain the implications of this research to my clients, a light goes on in their psyche, and they immediately understand what had been inexplicable for years.

The research on genes points clearly to the importance of smart food strategies. It has implications for appetite and weight control, shopping, how you display food, and where you keep it in your house. However, remember one thing: *Genes impel; they don't compel.* And with smart food-management strategies, you can take control of the food, your genetic influence, and your weight. This chapter doesn't just explain why you may have found yourself repeatedly gaining back the same weight with the same foods. It sets the stage for appreciating the importance of the strategies to come, such as boxing it in, which will teach you to keep your favorite foods in your life and be in control of them—rather than letting them control you.

(Individuals in psychotherapy for psychological issues related to compulsive eating should not discontinue their therapy, but should bring this research to the attention of their therapist, so that this therapy may yield a more complete and permanent result.)

Lastly, it has great implications for your maintenance program, because even once you lose the weight, that doesn't mean you've lost the genetic sensitivity to the sight, taste, and smell of your trigger foods. And if you get sloppy about the structure of your eating habits and strategies, as many people do once they have lost the weight, you'll end up out of control again. More people have ended up fat again and again not because they're failing, but because they are failing to plan. When reading this chapter, you realize how one commandment builds on the other: that the structure of your eating habits as well as the types of food, the timing, and the situation (whether you eat certain types of food on an empty stomach or a full stomach) are critical variables that may either have never been discussed before or were simply ignored. They may be the foundation stone for determining your success at weight control and whether you'll be constantly hungry and have cravings or find it easy to succeed.

We can't change our basic genetic response to food, but we can alter it powerfully through strategy. Whether we control it or it controls us is up to us, through the power of these techniques.

One of the most powerful lessons I have learned from the failures of thousands of people at weight control is not *that those who fail have no willpower. It is that they had no structure for their eating.*

The Fourth Thin Commandment:
Structure Gives Control

COMMANDMENT ESSENTIALS

- Eat a snack with protein and fiber between 3 and 5 P.M.
- Always bring your own healthy snack to a meeting.
- Put together a "ThinPack," and never leave home without it.
- Do your food shopping right after breakfast or right after eating.
- Don't clip coupons.
- Stay away from food "minis," such as minimuffins, minibagels, and minicookies.
- At buffets and cocktail parties, use the smallest plate to serve yourself.

HAVE YOU EVER WONDERED WHY everybody swears by the latest diet, and you often end up knowing quite a few people who lose weight on it? You may have tried a few different diets yourself and found that each time you started a new one, you began dropping weight too.

What is the key ingredient that makes any diet work at the beginning, even though they are so different in their menu plans?

What all diets have in common is *structure*. They all achieve weight loss because they give you a blueprint for eating. Is there a diet in the world that doesn't tell you to eat three good meals every day plus a healthy snack in the afternoon? That *structure* reins in eating behavior that has been out of control.

So why do the vast majority of people who lose weight on diets fail to maintain that weight loss?

When dieters are taught to focus exclusively on calories and carbs, they don't see anything wrong with fiddling with the structure of their diets. They are led to believe that all that really matters is the "calorie budget." My client Paula was doing beautifully on her diet until she went back to skipping breakfast because that was her history from childhood. She began "making up" the calories with pizza for lunch. Similarly, Sandra eliminated her midafternoon snack, figuring she'd "lay away" those 200 calories and "spend" them on dessert after dinner. Ed started his diet by studying low-calorie menu plans and prepared all his meals at home. Three weeks later, when he'd lost enough weight to wear his tennis shorts without embarrassment, he went back to eating at his favorite all-you-can-eat buffet restaurant, figuring he could just as easily find low-calorie foods for his plate so it wouldn't be a problem.

The standard diets actually encourage people to play around with the diet, yet they fail to teach you the right *strategies* to keep you from returning to out-of-school eating. They don't help you see *the critical connection between structure and weight control*.

THE WALL STREET EATING SYNDROME

I discovered the critical relationship between structure and weight control by accident. Since I do my work in New York City, I have an unusually large number of clients who work on Wall Street. The lives of these busy people are characterized by extraordinary focus and accomplishment. Many have reached the top of one of the toughest professions in the world, and they did it in one of the toughest cities in the world. Yet each one of them had a long history of failure on weight programs—so plainly, the problem wasn't willpower!

Clark was the model of the successful Wall Street executive when he became my client: He had a top-floor office overlooking the Statue of Liberty and a wonderful home in the suburbs. He also epitomized the collection of eating habits I now call the Wall Street Eating Syndrome: Breakfast was a doughnut or a bagel with coffee that Clark grabbed at the train station on his way to work; when he was running late, he missed breakfast completely. Lunch for Clark was whatever was quickest. Sometimes he'd just grab a bag of cashews or a mere 90-calorie cup of yogurt he "borrowed" from his assistant. Then if he felt hungry because of having eaten too little, he would nibble on whatever snack foods were around the office or in the conference rooms. Most days, Clark waited until the New York Stock Market closed at 3 P.M. to eat his lunch, then he bolted down a hero sandwich or whatever food he could find in the company kitchen on his floor. Some days, he just kept picking on whatever was left over from meetings in the conference room.

Clark often had to entertain business associates after work, and if he was sitting at a bar having a beer, he'd eat all the crunchy things in the snack bowl. If he met people at a restaurant, he'd demolish the breadbasket before he ordered. On the evenings he headed directly home after work, Clark bought a hot pretzel while he waited for his train, if it was winter; in summer, he bought ice cream. When he finally walked into his house around 7 P.M., Clark devoured the leftovers from his kids' dinner or anything else he could get his hands on in the fridge while he waited to sit down with his wife for their dinner.

I once pointed out to Clark that during the day, he's so busy with his work that he can't stop to eat, and from 4 o'clock on, he can't stop eating.

After hearing similar stories of missed meals, grabbing food on the run, indiscriminate snacking, and uncontrolled eating before and after dinner from others who *didn't* work on Wall Street, I realized that the Wall Street Eating Syndrome is actually a mirror of what is happening to society as a whole. We are shifting away from being a society that sits down to meals three times a day. Instead, people eat in motion. Most critically, breakfast and lunch are about grabbing whatever is quickest—or those meals are simply skipped entirely. Around 3 o'clock, just like the bell that rings on Wall Street to close the market, a hunger bell rings inside people, and they start eating! Typically, people start grabbing whatever is around when their hunger gets too strong to ignore. They eat very quickly, so the food is not adequately digested, and the body is never really satisfied by the meal. There are very few calories taken in during the early part of the day, and there is excessive calorie consumption from the late afternoon into the evening. Whenever a person is running short on time, time is "borrowed" from breakfast or lunch. The quality or healthfulness of food is always secondary to how quickly it can be consumed. And a disproportionate amount of calories come from mindless nibbling on whatever food is around or from snack foods. There is little meal planning. There is even less *structure*.

WHAT IS STRUCTURE?

The structure of your eating habits is made up of these major components:

The timing and frequency of your meals

- Do you have established times to eat, and do you stick with them?
- Do you wait until you are hungry to eat?
- Do you skip any meals or replace them with snacks?
- Do you eat very quickly?

The type of meal you eat

- Is it a real meal or a quick snack in place of a meal?
- Is it adequate to carry you through the day?

How your home food shopping gets done

- What time of the day does it get done?
- What is bought?

The way your meals are served

- Buffet or family style?
- Or individually plated?
- Do you eat meals standing up or while traveling?

Your eating structure is either a bridge to control or it promotes failure in weight loss. People with weight problems are most often people who have *no* structure at all in the critical areas of eating behavior.

It's especially important that you begin by making sure that the timing, frequency, and quality of your meals and snacks are structured to promote weight loss. This is what I mean:

- Eat breakfasts and lunches that contain sufficient protein and fiber, even if they must be quick meals that you eat while you multitask.
- Eat a snack with both protein and fiber between 3 and 5 P.M.
- Don't go longer than 3 to 4 hours without a healthy meal or snack.
- Eat a dinner that contains a generous amount of high-fiber vegetables, a salad, and an adequate protein.
- *Never skip meals or snacks!*

The Worldwide Eating Syndrome?

Nutritionists in America have long puzzled over the so-called French Paradox or Italian Mystery because the French and Italian diets are so much richer in butters and cheeses than the American diet, yet the French and Italians have less obesity-related disease than Americans do. What researchers have overlooked is that eating in France and Italy has long been *structured* into three meals a day, with an afternoon course of fruit or small cheese—with snacking being discouraged.

People in these countries do not skip meals (although Italians eat them later than we do). Random snacking is very rare. (Children are not given free rein with the refrigerator and microwave.) If you look into the pantry of an Italian or French kitchen, it is not loaded with the junk food you see in American homes. Heavy desserts are reserved for holidays and special occasions. Europeans shop almost daily for fresh foods that they use completely in making one meal—as opposed to bringing enough food into the house each week to stock an air-raid shelter. It's neither a paradox nor a mystery: It's *structure!*

(It's an interesting commentary that most of my European clients would consider it a form of child abuse to feed their children or keep in the home all that junk food that many American clients are convinced their children can't live without. Perhaps that is the only paradox.)

I have discovered that most of my weight clients skip either breakfast or lunch—and sometimes both—or eat inadequately at those meals. But almost no one ever skips dinner. Indeed, dinner is the meal where most people overconsume. Having seen the weight gains this lack of structure has caused in my clients, I am most concerned that you eat a proper breakfast and lunch so that you don't get too hungry as the day wears on and fall into the Wall Street Eating Syndrome.

The diet and menu section of this book is filled with specific suggestions for the ideal quick breakfast and lunch as well as delicious dinners. They may not take long to consume, but they will keep you satisfied and energetic. You will also find plenty of information about what constitutes a healthy snack, including brand-name ingredients that are easy to find and are portable.

NEVER LET A DIET MAKE YOU HUNGRY

The very biggest mistake any dieter can make is to skip meals or go too long without food. There is as much danger in eating too little when you are trying to lose weight as eating too much. If you let yourself become hungry, you will feel compelled to eat whatever you see first, and you will eat compulsively—or you'll be living with constant feelings of being deprived. Your own body has its own structure for eating, and unless the structure of your eating mirrors the body's structure, your weight can spin out of control.

Feeling hungry is not a sign that you are virtuously following your diet.

Feeling hungry is a sure sign that your diet is wrong or your eating habits are wrong.

We have a wealth of scientific studies that show that people who eat small nutritious meals frequently do much better with weight control than people who eat big meals infrequently. It's easy enough to see why: From your body's point of view, the very purpose of eating is to avoid hunger. If you do not feed your body adequate calories every 3 or 4 hours, then the next time you eat anything, you will set off a chemical chain reaction inside your body that makes you compulsively eat more.

What do I mean when I say "adequate calories?" Your breakfast and lunch should be made up of foods that have enough nutrients to carry you through your busy day to the next meal without getting hungry. A single cup of fat-free yogurt, for instance, is an excellent snack food, but it's not sufficient as a lunch by itself. If you look at the meal plans in this book, you will see that the structure of your meal should be built around providing your body with sufficient protein, fiber, and other nutrients so that you are never hungry.

Some people tell me that when they are "in the zone" to lose weight, it doesn't bother them to skip meals. But I have found that over a period of weeks, this skipping of meals invariably leads to cheating and losses of control with eating. Of all the thousands of people I've worked with, I can think of very few, if any, who skip meals on a regular basis and who kept their weight off. Perhaps that will convince you how important not skipping is.

Structure Is the Cravings Killer

There is another important reason why you should never go too long without eating. Almost all cravings come from what I call "The Four S's": Seeing, Smelling, Stress, and Starvation. In combination, the "Four S's" throw a lethal curve at your ability to control what you eat. We are powerfully guided by our senses, which is a fact known to every modern advertiser and supermarket owner. They do everything they can to keep food in front of your eyes or get you to turn your head to look at it. And if they can get you to smell it when you're hungry, that's even better!

Structure Right Now

One of the best ways to immediately structure your eating and shopping habits is to start keeping a food diary (see page 162), like the one I use with my own clients, which guides and reinforces structure. Studies on weight control indicate that people lose more weight when they keep a diary while on a weight program.

THE FOURTH THIN COMMANDMENT

By giving yourself a solid structure of frequent meals and snacks every day, you protect yourself against the siren songs of the Four S's. It's simply a physiological fact that if you go too long without eating, your blood sugar falls, and you are more prone to feel stressed and irritable. You may not be aware that you are setting yourself up to be overcome by cravings, since your mind is preoccupied with the activities of the day. But as soon as you encounter the sight or smell of a food that you like, it will have an impact on your appetite that is a thousand times more powerful than if you encountered those same foods on a full stomach. Your chances of being selective about what you eat and the amount you eat now are almost nonexistent!

As C. Wayne Calloway, M.D., an endocrinologist at George Washington University, has observed, when you wait until you feel hungry before you eat, you jump-start the production of neuropeptide Y, which can lead to uncontrollable cravings, especially for carbohydrates. And once that happens, it's like losing the brake on your appetite, and you become "an eating automaton."

Arthur Agatston, M.D., the famed author of *The South Beach Diet,* has warned that "the carbohydrates that dominate the typical American diet—white bread, pasta, cereal, snack foods, cakes, cookies, candies, and so on—are stripped of fiber during processing. These foods are quickly digested and absorbed as glucose, the form sugar takes in the bloodstream. The body must produce increasing amounts of insulin to remove excess glucose in the blood." Not only does this dangerously promote the storage of fat around the abdomen, Dr. Agatston points out, "high insulin levels end up removing too much glucose from the blood. The resulting low-blood sugar, called reactive hypoglycemia, triggers food cravings. The more you give in to your cravings, the more weight you gain."

If you go too long without eating and then you turn to these simple carbohydrates, you feel you are out of control with your appetite and your eating—you may even find yourself bingeing. This is a physiological phenomenon that many people incorrectly interpret as a psychological, emotional eating disorder. In truth, the disorder is completely physiological, caused by the lack of structure in your eating habits combined with the excessive consumption of simple carbohydrates.

ENDING FOOD CRAVINGS FOREVER

The best way to keep cravings from ruining your diet is to prevent them. Preventing anything in this world from happening, especially anything with a lot of history of occurring, requires planning and strategy. Prevention is preferable to rehabilitation, and it's much cheaper!

Planning and eating the right breakfast is the right strategy. Planning and eating the right lunch is the right strategy too. Both will keep you from having the feelings of hunger and dissatisfaction from cravings grow. Equally important: *Eating a healthy snack every afternoon is an essential strategy in the prevention of food cravings, because it keeps your blood sugar stable and keeps hunger at bay.*

Still Balking at Eating Breakfast?

Some of my clients tell me that eating breakfast when they get up makes them more, not less, hungry as the morning wears on. Most of these clients were eating the wrong type of breakfast: one with too much sugar or too little fiber—or both. The biggest culprits seem to be sugary flaked cereals, bagels, breakfast tarts, or even some kinds of oatmeal that are low in fiber (such as instant). If you have a history of becoming hungrier after eating breakfast, the first strategy to try is eating a *different kind of breakfast.* Experiment with the breakfast suggestions in the menu section of this book (see page 203), and focus on making a breakfast with protein. *Don't* skip breakfast altogether.

Some of my clients are simply never hungry when they get up. The answer for these people is to move their breakfast time to later in the morning, around 10:30 A.M. and then not eat lunch until 2 P.M. (The time of day is secondary, the structure of three meals and a snack sometime between lunch and dinner is primary.) Just make sure you always eat a breakfast. The universal laws of the human body require it.

The Cinderella Syndrome

Most of my clients suffer from what I call "the Cinderella Syndrome." For Cinderella, everything went south at midnight. For them, everything starts going south in the middle of the afternoon.

Within a few hours after eating lunch, usually around 4 P.M., most people's blood sugar starts to dip. Unless they head off hunger with a truly healthy snack, as blood sugar goes lower and lower, people who are carbohydrate abusers tend to find themselves craving sweets or flour products. If you give in to that craving for simple carbohydrates, you trigger a chaotic cycle of chemical ups-and-downs that, by the time dinnertime rolls around, will make you a compulsive eater instead of a selective one. If you find this craving cycle is a factor in your life, you can end it with two simple steps:

1. Remind yourself (if you're craving sweets or junk snacks): This is not about sweets or junk. It's 4 P.M., and my blood sugar is low. That's why I want something sweet.

2. Eat a low-fat protein snack such as a fat-free/low-fat yogurt with some fresh berries, or another low-sugar fruit or a protein with fiber such as my recommended low-fat cheese with the high-fiber bran crackers (such as Laughing Cow Light Cheese Triangles with GG Scandinavian Bran Crispbread). Other people find that an apple with one of the cheese triangles or a protein shake such as Alba, CarbSolutions, or EAS Carb Control works brilliantly.

YOUR THINPACK: NEVER LEAVE HOME WITHOUT IT!

Life is unpredictable. I teach my clients never to be without an extra healthy snack in their purse or briefcase. That's so they will never have to worry that they might lose to a cookie or a bag of peanuts when life throws them an unexpected curve ball, and their next meal is delayed. Having a smart food strategy means that you, too, will never succumb to eating the cookies at a conference or school event for your kids and that you will never grab fattening food on the run. It also means you will *never* be hungry.

Since we live in a very busy world, I've come up with a perfect way to guarantee that you'll never be battling cravings because you've gone too long without eating: a ThinPack!

What's a ThinPack?

It's a self-sealing bag that contains two or three high-fiber crackers (such as the GG Scandinavian Bran Crispbread or Bran-a-Crisp), an apple, and two low-fat, prewrapped cheese wedges (such as Mini-Bonbel or Laughing Cow), which can go for a few hours without refrigeration. If cheese is a trigger food for you, substitute slices of low-fat cold cuts or 2 tablespoons of peanut butter for a delicious sandwich with the crackers, or any other form of protein *that you have no history of abusing.* Shelled nuts are tricky for some, but Knight's Light or Weight Watcher's popcorn in a small bag provides a delicious, high-fiber substitute.

With your ThinPack right at hand at all times, you can weather any delay or unexpected change in your schedule.

Dinner after 7?

Many of my clients get into trouble because their partner gets home from work later than they do, and they become ravenously hungry waiting to eat dinner. Some end up eating their kids' food while they wait, others keep picking at the dinner ingredients, eating bread and snack foods, or they just don't eat anything and gorge at dinner.

If you aren't likely to have dinner within 4 hours of your afternoon snack, add an early evening snack to your daily menu plan, preferably one with protein and fiber, such as a small serving of cheese with an apple or bran crackers, or a tomato juice and celery with fat-free cream cheese. Or, for about the same number of calories, have a minimeal such as a shrimp cocktail, an egg-white omelet with vegetables, or a couple of scoops of my Dilled Egg Salad (see page 221).

We were wrongly told as children "Don't spoil your dinner!" when we reached for a snack while waiting for the adults to make supper. Since most weight clients consume the greatest amount of their calories around dinnertime, get rid of that outdated advice. Never go hungry to dinner. Don't worry about spoiling your appetite; worry about spoiling your figure or your weight loss!

THIN STARTS IN THE SUPERMARKET

I tell my clients that they should never walk into any type of grocery store, farmer's market, or specialty food store if they are hungry. (Eat first, and wait for the hunger to pass.) And never go shopping without a list. Wandering around a supermarket looking for things to buy almost guarantees that you will automatically buy many of the same foods that made you fat. Also, it only stimulates your curiosity to try new foods—on top of what already is tempting you. If you have a problem with snack foods or junk foods, it's not a good idea to go shopping with your children, because the packaging on many unhealthy foods is designed to attract a child's interest. You'll likely end up with a kitchen full of snack foods that will undermine your weight-loss program.

I also strongly discourage my clients from doing *any* food shopping after work. Most people are mentally fatigued and hungry at the end of the day, which means they're more likely to succumb to impulse buying when they are surrounded by the sights and smells of food. By contrast, very few people feel any urge to overeat in the morning.

The best time to go food shopping is right after breakfast or right after eating. The worst time is between 3 and 6 P.M. If you must shop at this time, eat a healthy snack first.

With a satisfied stomach, you'll be less tempted by the brightly colored, alluring packaging of junk foods and frozen desserts and the aromas of fresh baked goods.

My client Eva switched to doing her shopping on Sunday mornings after breakfast, and not only did she find the market less crowded than during the evening "rush hour," she more easily lost weight than she had before. Dorothy, who is a single mother, tried switching to shopping on Saturday mornings instead of doing it on her way home from work, but she discovered that her kids would want to go with her and then it was much harder to control what went into the shopping cart. Dorothy went back to shopping after work, but on her way to the market, she drinks a small can of V-8 juice and eats a sandwich made of bran crackers and low-fat cold cuts. Her shopping hours no longer interfere with her weight loss. Pick the strategy that works best for your weight loss. Just make sure you *never* enter a food store feeling hungry.

MEAL STRUCTURE AND THE "E.A.T. PRINCIPLE"

Your meals and snacks themselves can and should have a firm structure that optimizes your control over eating. Buffets and all-you-can-eat restaurants offer only *unstructured* eating. So do Chinese restaurants and dining "family style" at home (where everybody serves themselves from large dishes that are passed around the table). Snacking directly from a supersize bag of popcorn or picking over

Shopping with Structure

Before you take your next trip to the store, review these tips, and keep them in mind as you're walking up and down the aisles.

Beware the "bargain size"! People who buy bargain-size bags of food get no bargain at all. They end up spending the few pennies they save on larger-size clothing and, far worse, doctor's bills and prescription medications.

Buy your food in structures that help you eat less. Buy as much of your food as you can packaged in units that minimize the possibility of your over-consuming or having any leftovers from your meal or your snack. People always eat less when presented with individualized servings and tend to eat much more from large bags and boxes.

Don't clip coupons. Most of the foods aggressively marketed with coupons that arrive as inserts in our Sunday newspaper are high-fat foods or

plain old junk foods that have no place in your diet. Don't be tempted to buy a food just because you have a coupon for it or because you've never tried it before.

Stick to your list. Always make a shopping list before you enter a food store, even if you have to stand outside the door and write one up. Inside the store, *stick to your list!* You don't need a food just because it's on sale. Yes, over time, you wind up paying a few dollars more at the cash register each week when you live inside a good structure, but you get a priceless payoff in good health and a happier life.

Don't buy foods for others that you have a history of abusing, unless they specifically ask for them. If they do, buy the smallest size possible, and ask them to keep it out of your sight. If you do buy snack foods for others, buy ones that are not your favorites to reduce temptation.

an entire bunch of grapes on the kitchen counter is also eating without structure. Eating foods and meals without structure is a prelude to excessive consumption and losses of control.

Through my work with thousands of weight clients, I have discovered what I consider to be something close to a law of human nature. I call it "E.A.T." or the Expanding Appetite Theorem: *Appetite expands to consume the amount of food presented.* If you are served 4 ounces of food, you will eat 4 ounces of food. If you are served 8 ounces, you will eat 8 ounces. If you go to buffets or family-style restaurants, you will eat more than if you go to a restaurant where all your food is put on a plate for you alone by the chef. If you buy the largest bag of popcorn at the market or the movies, you will eat far more popcorn than if you buy the smallest.

But I've also discovered that there is an equal force in nature that opposes E.A.T.: *The more precisely structured your food is, the less likely you are to overeat it.* An example? You will always eat only one serving of potato if it's baked, but you may not know when to stop if it's mashed. Similarly, people will often eat far less calories in a restaurant if they order a baked potato with their entrée instead of rice. One restaurant serving of rice can be anything from half a cup to half a plateful, and most people will finish all that is served to them. The larger portion does not give any greater sense of satiety of satisfaction than the smaller one does. We simply eat the extra amount just because it's there.

Have You Got Unophobia?

I've noticed that hundreds, perhaps even thousands, of my clients feel deprived and depressed if they see one lonely piece of anything on their plate, whether it is one slice of bread or an egg. But they instantly cheer up if their food has a mate. If you're a "unophobic," cut your serving into two pieces! It's amazing how much more satisfied people feel eating two halves of a peach instead of a whole one or one hard-boiled egg that's been sliced into quarters. Similarly, you'll be much more satisfied with two pieces of 40-calorie light wheat bread than with one piece of the regular wheat bread for 80 calories.

The same applies to fresh fruits you eat for a dessert or snack. Have you ever eaten more than one apple at a time? But you're likely to eat too many cherries or pineapple chunks if you dish them out of a big bowl or can. In the summer, many of my clients have seen their weight loss stop or diminish because they keep bowls of cut-up fruit in the refrigerator and overeat it constantly.

People eat with their eyes as much as they eat with their mouths. The larger the serving or the availability, the more you will eat. I strongly advise my clients to run away from the food "minis": minimuffins, minibagels, minicookies, and even minifruits such as lady apples, prune plums, or mandarin oranges.

It seems that many of my male clients don't realize that, at social events, they eat far more calories during the cocktail hour picking at bite-size finger foods (such as pigs-in-a-blanket) than they eat during the entire dinner itself. The food "minis" either fool you into believing you're barely eating at all or that you can't be eating too many calories, since the serving size is so small. And they make it too easy for you to lose count of how much you're eating.

If you eat like the intelligent people who sit in my office, you'll consume more calories eating the "minis" than you would have had you simply served yourself one normal portion of food. (The only exception I make to my "anti-mini" rule is low-fat minicheeses that are individually sealed in wax or foil. Dieters are less likely to overeat these premeasured servings that have to be unwrapped than if they try to slice 1 ounce of cheese from a block. The cheese block becomes like the bowl of cut-up fruit. People keep going back for instant, repeat servings.)

STRUCTURE EMPOWERS YOU TO DO THE RIGHT THING

Structure prevents the cravings and hunger that tempt you to violate your diet. It guides you in planning your meals and snacks and your food shopping. It guides you to being protective of yourself and honoring your body's needs. *When people structure their eating habits, within a week or two they feel back in control of their life again.* By eating at regular intervals, your *hunger* has dissipated, and your crav-

Strategies for Buffets, Family-Style Restaurants, All-You-Can-Eat Restaurants, and Cocktail Parties

Here are some hints and tips to put into action when you know you're going to be faced with a lot of food in a social setting.

Eat a snack before you go out to eat or to a party.

Say to yourself before you walk in: "I've seen it all and tasted it all before; there's nothing really new. It's glorified cafeteria food."

Put Listerine Breath Strips on your tongue before you enter to block the tempting aromas.

Drink a glass of tomato juice or a Virgin Bloody Mary when you arrive.

Do not survey the entire buffet.

Pick the smallest plate or a child's plate to serve yourself, not an oversize dinner plate.

Say to yourself before you put any food on your plate: "If I eat it all, I will wear it all."

Take only one main entrée or two half servings of entrées. Then go directly to the vegetable and salad section. Avoid vegetables or salads sitting in oil or butter.

Strive to make your plate look like a regular restaurant plate of food.

Don't survey the dessert section if desserts are your issue.

Say to yourself after you've eaten one serving: "It's more important to get my life's worth than my money's worth."

At a cocktail party or standing buffet, carry a clutch purse plus a beverage, or a cup and saucer. If your hands are full, you can't eat.

---

ings have dissipated, even though you are eating a fraction of the calories your were eating before.

You no longer feel like a failure, and why should you ever?

Structure is not only part of a successful *diet*. It must remain part of a successful eating style. The reason so many people succeed at weight loss but fail at weight maintenance is that once their clothes fit better, they get loose with structure. And once they are loose about structure, they fall back into the throes of old cravings and temptations. This is a certainty, so if you want lasting success, remember: *Structure gives control—and structure guards control.*

Happy or sad, rich or poor . . . it's still better being thin.
Even if you want to be miserable today, it's better to be
thin and miserable than fat and miserable.

The Fifth Thin Commandment:

Separate Mood from Food

COMMANDMENT ESSENTIALS

- Don't buy snacks you habitually abuse when you are stressed.
- Keep tempting snack foods (that you must have on hand for family members) out of sight.
- Keep healthy snack foods available.
- Pick up the phone, and chat with a friend instead of picking up a chip or cookie.
- Practice yoga, weed your garden, knit, or do some other activity instead of stress eating.
- Switch to a stress food substitute that won't make you fat.
- Talk yourself out of mood eating.

SOMETIMES EATING IS NOT about food.

Emotional eating is one of the most pervasive and overwhelming issues for dieters to deal with. It's also one of the most insidious, because no matter how much weight you lose, if the next time you get upset, you return to your old ways, your castle is built on sand.

Diets that focus on caloric thinking have no answers for people who have a history of mood eating. They offer no strategies to block it or end it. As long as we approach dieting with an oversimplified model of calories in and calories out, the very high failure rate for dieters will remain what it is because we have lost sight of the human being who is the most important factor in the equation. In dealing with a human behavior, one plus one often does not equal two. There is logic—and there is *psycho*logic.

At the opposite extreme, unfortunately, most discussions of mood eating are overloaded with psychobabble. Since I have a background in a branch of psychology that explores human motivation rather than psychopathology, I didn't enter the field of weight control with a belief that just because a person has gained weight, he must have some hidden psychological problem. As I have said before, *We don't have to be crazy to be crazy about a cookie!*

The obvious reason that people use a food to change their mood is that the food they are abusing *tastes* good. Almost all mood eaters reach for snacks with a sweet taste or creamy texture, or they want a crunchy texture that is salty or sweet. Those tastes and textures provide mood eaters with *immediate satisfaction.* Crunching on something may actually relieve pent-up emotions in the same way pummeling a pillow would. And when you keep lots of such snack foods around your house, eating to spill your emotions becomes more user-friendly and immediate.

I will never tell you that the foods you choose to eat as mood lifters don't have a pleasurable taste. They do. But nothing tastes better than looking in the mirror every morning and feeling proud of what you see. Food pleasure is fleeting, and I've yet to meet the stress eater who is happy with his behavior or himself for doing it!

Mood eating is a learned behavior, and fortunately, whatever has been learned can be unlearned, even if we learned it long ago and have strengthened the lessons through habit. The good news is that even though mood eating is one of the most pervasive and insidious challenges faced by dieters and traditional weight-control programs, it is one of the most amenable to correct through strategy. When you look closely at actual histories of mood eaters, you make a liberating discovery.

For the overwhelming majority, mood eating isn't about food—and it's not about fine dining. It's about snacking and grabbing whatever is around in your immediate environment that looks "interesting."

My client Sonia loves to cook, but when she gets stressed, she doesn't drop everything to bake her favorite lasagna. She'll just raid her kids' cookie jar. Craig truly enjoys gourmet food, but when he has a lousy day at the office, he doesn't slip into a fine restaurant and order three main courses. He'll eat a large-size bag of chips on his way home. Marilyn's New York apartment is right down the street from an all-night gourmet food store, but every time she gets an aggravating phone call from her sister, she'll only binge on ice cream as long as she doesn't have to walk one step farther than the fridge to get it!

So the pattern is clear: Mood eating isn't about food. It's about snacking and grabbing whatever is around. *Mood eating is about immediacy—right now.*

What mood eaters want is an *immediate* change in their feelings. That's why it's about *snacking,* not real food, and it's about snacking on what's easiest to get into your mouth. In all the years I've been working on weight control in the most stress-ridden city in America, the number of clients I've had who reacted to stress by cooking, shopping, or dining in restaurants is so small that, while I can't say I can count the number on the fingers of two hands, I don't need many more fingers than that. I've worked successfully with thousands of stress eaters, and despite their sex differences, and diverse backgrounds, and economic status, I would estimate that close to 90 percent shared this single common pattern when it came to mood eating:

• **Same food.** Mood eaters return time and time again to their favorite snack food—a snack that is either crunchy (such as chips, crackers, pretzels, or even cereal); sweet (such as cookies and candies); or creamy (such as ice cream or frozen yogurt). Most typically, they prefer a bite-size food that they can keep popping into their mouths, almost independent of whether they are hungry or not.

• **Same place.** Mood eaters eat alone in the kitchen. A very small number do their mood eating at their office.

• **Same time of day.** Mood eating is done in the late afternoon or evening, almost never in the morning.

• **Same moods.** It's feelings of anxiety, anger, frustration, betrayal, disappointment, or boredom that are the common triggers for mood eating.

• **Same people.** Mood eaters snack because they become stressed by the same *people* over and over again (such as a boss, a partner, a child, a relative, or a friend).

• **Same situations.** Mood eaters snack because they become stressed by the same *situations* over and over again (such as having to make presentations at work or being in uncomfortable social situations), or they're bored, and eating becomes "something interesting to do."

• **Same quantities of food.** Mood eating is almost always about volume. Whether one is dealing with frustration or boredom, a mood doesn't evaporate with one M&M. As the mood lingers, people want the eating to linger also, so they choose snacks with a "long-eating" time—like a bag of M&Ms.

• **Same reason.** Mood eaters want a treat or comfort from the

Are You a Boredom Eater?

One of the surprising things I've discovered about boredom eaters is that, unlike other mood eaters, the act of snacking is more important to them than what they snack on. While most mood eaters aren't really happy unless they can munch their favorite snacks, boredom eaters will eat anything so long as it fills up time, and they can easily pick at it from the kitchen counter, the refrigerator, or cabinets.

Planning is the cure for boredom eating. Designing a flower bed, reading an interesting book, sending e-mails to your friends, or just about any activity you can think of that's legal is a better use of your time than boredom eating!

But even the most organized people can end up with unstructured time on their hands. If you are a boredom eater, keep a plate of raw vegetables in your refrigerator or a single bag of light popcorn you can chew on. Especially avoid bringing home the fascinating finger food you see in the market, like nuts and flavored crackers, and never use food shopping as an escape from tedium. When simple boredom turns into high-fat boredom eating, people can end up literally bored to death.

food. That is why mood eating is almost always done with a food they buy and bring home for themselves, even if they may believe they bought it for others, especially their family or company.

If you're a frequent mood eater, there's a very good chance that you do it because of the same moods caused by the same people and same situations that caused you stress before, and you do your mood eating alone in the same place, at the same time of day, and with the same food nearly every time.

Once you realize your mood eating is totally predictable, you can control it with strategy!

Judy was an extremely intelligent hospital executive who came to me after a number of therapists failed to help her control her mood eating. "Why do I keep doing this," she asked angrily in my office, "when I know I'm just eating out of stress and tension? I'm not even hungry!" As I asked her questions about her eating patterns, it became clear that Judy always made a beeline for any kind of sweet, baked good that was also a finger food, such as cookies or baked minimuffins. She never went for the snacks her husband had around the house, because she didn't like his salty, crunchy foods.

I couldn't help but ask Judy, "Why do you keep buying *your* type of snack food and bringing it home when you know you're a mood eater?"

THE BEST PLACE TO END
MOOD EATING FOREVER

The best place to end mood eating is not a psychiatrist's couch. It's the supermarket. If you know you have a tendency to eat when you are upset, don't buy the snacks you habitually abuse when you are stressed or bring them into the house because your own kitchen is probably where you do most of your mood eating.

The interesting and even wonderful thing about ending the pattern of mood eating is that when snacks aren't immediately available, almost all mood eaters automatically busy themselves with a *noneating* activity, such as watching TV, listening to music, or cleaning out a closet, which disperses their energy. In the end, no matter what the burdens and stresses of your life may be, you can't eat what's not there! But mood eaters can't get beyond compulsive snacking if they keep their kitchen stocked with convenient snacks.

Once Judy scratched all the snack foods off her shopping list, she was astonished that her mood eating disappeared, and her subsequent weight loss was significant. "I never dreamed I could do it so easily," she marveled 2 months later, by which time she was already one dress size smaller. Judy had become even more fit by putting a Ping-Pong table in her basement to work out her stresses with her kids.

Buying or having your favorite snack foods in the house encourages and reinforces the destructive habit of mood eating. I've learned that quite a few of my clients are like Peter, who works from home as a computer consultant. It used to be that whenever Peter had peanut M&Ms in his house, he magnified every minor setback that came along during the day into an excuse to eat. When his Internet connection went down, when a delivery didn't arrive, Peter decided he "needed" a snack break. Peter does most of the family shopping, and he insisted that the only reason he bought the family-size bags of peanut M&Ms was because his kids ate them too. But his kids almost never saw any of them! Peter switched to buying Fruit Rollups for his kids and stopped bringing peanut M&Ms into the house, and his own "stress" snacking stopped. He not only lost his spare tire, Peter claims he has the best-organized home office in Connecticut!

Strategies for Snack Foods

If you know your favorite nibble is right in the next room, the least provocation or annoyance can become the excuse to indulge. The very availability of the snack creates conscious and unconscious rationalizations to keep on eating it.

Why not employ a strategy right now, and toss out the "mood snacks" that are in your kitchen? When you make up your next shopping list, simply don't add those foods to your list—and while you are in the market, please stick to your list. If someone else does the family shopping, ask for their cooperation in making you trim.

If you absolutely must keep snacks in your home for other people, here are proven strategies to keep you from eating them:

• Ask others in your home for permission to buy a type of snack that is not your favorite or that you are unlikely to abuse. If they insist on having a snack that tempts you, buy only a single serving that's just for them, and give it to them immediately to keep. (It's always a smart strategy to buy *all* snacks in single, individually wrapped servings, because snacks are a type of food that is so easy to overconsume.)

• Keep snack foods out of sight. Take all snack foods out of their highly attractive packaging, and keep them in plain brown bags or containers that aren't transparent. Another good strategy is to keep snacks behind a cupboard door that you rarely open or that is out of your line of vision, or keep them at the back of your most hard-to-reach shelf. *Never keep snacks on the kitchen counter.* It encourages mindless snacking. The kitchen counter is the single most dangerous spot in your house for your weight-control efforts. It's easily accessible, and it's the first thing people see and reach for (whether they are hungry or not) when there is food on it.

• Ask those in your immediate family and your good friends not to snack in front of you whenever possible.

• Have family members hide tempting snack foods if you're given to grazing.

• If nothing else works, lock all snacks in a cash box with a combination lock, and make sure only those who eat the snacks enclosed have the combination.

• Keep healthy snack foods available (like an apple or cut-up vegetables), so you're not tempted to go on to the fattening ones.

Remember: Living your life trim and healthy is far more important than spending extra money on a lockbox or worrying that a strategy looks "crazy." The only thing that's crazy is your looking fat because you're going down the tubes again and again for snack food!

When we dispense with the need to be normal, life gets so much easier! I am convinced that one of the reasons my clients are so successful at losing weight and keeping it off is that they are able to think outside the box. They quickly learn not to ask: "Is this normal?" They just respect what works. What works for you *is* what's normal for your life!

IS IT REALLY A CRISIS?

Carl was a longtime client of mine whose beloved father had a stroke. Carl spent entire days and nights at the hospital, and I only learned of the situation when Carl's wife called me to say that she was alarmed because Carl had eaten very little for days. Despite his long history of mood eating, Carl is like most of us: When we are profoundly upset, we lose our appetite.

It's actually the *day-to-day annoyances,* not the profound upsets, that prompt mood eaters to reach for their snacks. Almost all mood eating is really about simply getting rid of a stressful day or event. It's about immediately substituting a pleasurable feeling for an un-pleasant one. That's why when the shock of a genuine crisis hits us, it never occurs to us to open up a bag of chips.

The key to controlling mood eating is recognizing that the vast majority of the time, the kind of stress that does make us want to eat is *predictable* stress: It is stress that comes from the same familiar people and the same familiar situations time and time again.

Strategies for Stress on the Horizon

If your youngest child is starting kindergarten next week; if your older brother spoils every family occasion, and your parents' 40th anniversary is coming up; if you'll have to deliver last quarter's dis-appointing sales report to management on Thursday, you have every reason in the world to plan in advance what you are going to eat on those days. One day of stress really doesn't have to become a legacy of fat.

When stress looms, I have found that three simple techniques dramatically reduce the likelihood of your turning to food to relieve the stress:

Write out what you will eat for that day in advance. Create a sample menu for what you will eat for breakfast, lunch, dinner, and snacks. Direct your psyche to think in terms of these foods only and to avoid all others.

Plan which snacks you are going to eat, and keep all others out of sight. (When making up your ThinPack, you probably want the items for a predictable "stress day" to have some crunch.)

Plan to avoid trouble. Don't drive down a road that takes you past your favorite bakery on a day when you know you'll be stressed out. Take all the change out of your pockets before you walk to the conference room if you know you'll have to pass the vending machines.

I've almost always found that when people plan what they're going to eat on a "stress day" and how they're going to stay away from trouble, they're able to get through any stressful situation successfully.

Give Your Stress a Dress Rehearsal

Many mood-eating clients find it very helpful to mentally rehearse what they expect to encounter from a stressful person or situation. If it's a person who is surely going to give you trouble, you can tell yourself: "I know what she is going to say and how she's going to react." You can rehearse the words you fear hearing in your own mind until they lose their power to provoke you. Also rehearse what you will say or do in response. Mentally walking yourself through a dreaded situation several times in advance can dispel a lot of anxiety and make you feel confident of your ability to control the situation, including your eating.

A WINNER ALWAYS PLANS FOR THE UNKNOWN

We all know not every stressful day is predictable. Life happens! It has curveballs. Even when you already know that it's mainly your kids or coworkers who cause you to feel stressed, you can't always predict *when* a day that begins as a breeze will snowball into disaster. Your kids don't plan to break expensive lamps. Your coworkers don't plan to make the computer system crash. The winners at weight control don't let the unknown catch them unprepared.

"Planning is stronger than willpower!" is the motto that all my former mood eaters live by. They've come to appreciate the beauty of planning in keeping stress from turning into fat!

You can join them in the winner's circle of weight control by making their winning strategies your own. If you haven't done it already, make a list of your friends' telephone numbers, so you can dial them easily when stress next hits. Decide right now that the next time you feel a bad mood rising, you'll spend a few minutes with a favorite activity, especially one that occupies your hands. (Ex-smokers in particular should look for ways to keep their hands busy, so they don't start picking at fattening finger foods.)

My client Daniel throws darts at a wooden bull's-eye that he hung on the back of his office door. Alice's ongoing project is to arrange her CD collection into perfect order. (You can listen to music while you do it!) Laura sorts through her vacation photos and puts them into albums. If you have a drawer at home or in your office that's become a catch-all, you might promise yourself that the next time you're upset, you'll straighten out that drawer.

A reader of *More* magazine recently wrote to its editors to say: "When I pick up my knitting, I feel an instantaneous physical response. My blood pressure drops and I experience a calmness throughout my body. Knitting is my yoga!"

If you're a mood eater, it's wise to find *your* yoga! (Maybe yoga *is* your yoga!) If you don't have a healthy, constructive outlet for stress, look for one you'd like to adopt. Focus on activities that you can do at home that don't require an elaborate setup, so you'll be able to turn to them immediately. Try to avoid activities that are so demanding that they might frustrate you or increase your stress. And make sure the activity you choose interests you enough that boredom doesn't tempt you to eat!

Best Activities to Block Stress Eating

Don't let stress get the better of you and your weight. The next time you feel stressed out, try one of these activities instead of heading for the kitchen.

Knitting and crocheting
Taking a warm bath or shower
Playing with a Game Boy
Playing with a pet
Saying a favorite prayer
Keeping a diary
Sending e-mails to friends
Going online to learn about something that interests you
Having sex
Stretching and exercising, especially with hand weights
Meditation or yoga
Squeezing a rubber ball
Watching a video or reading a compelling book
Playing an instrument
Shopping for items you enjoy (other than food)

IF YOU CAN'T STOP IT, SWITCH IT

In a perfect world, I would tell you that the best way to rid yourself of your stress is to always stop what you are doing, exercise vigorously, or take a warm bath. Science suggests this is the best route, but sometimes—in fact, most times—life doesn't give us this opportunity.

My client Nancy is a mood eater who told me before I'd even offered her a list of strategies that she didn't have the time or energy for diversions when she's stressed out. Nancy has toddler twins and a 5-year-old who keep her running in three different directions every minute of the day. By the time she manages to get them all to sleep each night, the only thing Nancy can think about doing is curling up in an easy chair with a magazine and cookies. She'd keep eating cookies as she read, and she'd end up eating as many as a dozen.

We all have to work with the way our lives really are, not the way other people tell us they should be. My job is to help my clients stay trim without asking them to enter monasteries or submit to personality transplants. *One of my great surprises was to learn that most stress eaters are very open to switching to foods that have similar characteristics to the foods they abuse, but which aren't fattening. They will even feel better immediately if they switch to a food that is healthy for them.*

Typically, people are looking for just two things from their "stress" snack: They want it immediately at hand, and they want it to be pleasurable. So I suggested to Nancy that instead of snacking on cookies, she switch to whole grain waffles (such as Van's) and a diet hot chocolate. (I recommend Swiss Miss Diet or Carnation Diet.) The next time I saw her, Nancy told me she was delighted with the switch: The crunchy waffle was easy to make and delicious. Because of its high-fiber content, a whole grain waffle gave her enough of a feeling of satisfaction that it replaced all 12 cookies she had been eating. Nancy told me that the diet hot chocolate, which was only 25 calories, added an extra dimension of relaxation to the end of her day.

Crunch a Bunch of Healthy Snacks

Jack is a statistician who works for New York's department of public health, and he spends long hours in front of his computer, building

Stress Substitutes That Won't Make You Fat

If you absolutely have to reach for a snack when stressed, it doesn't have to be something that's going to add on the pounds. Here's a quick glance at the foods that spell trouble in times of stress—and healthy substitutes that won't sabotage your diet.

The Dangers

Cookies, especially small ones

Chocolates

Chewy candies such as gummy bears

Crunchy *thin* crackers that are salty and flavorful (especially Triscuits and Wheat Thins)

Crunchy or sweetened cereals, such as granola and raisin bran squares

Chips

Pretzels

Mounds of cheese you can keep picking on or baked "cheese sticks"

Nuts and trail mixes

Finger fruits such as grapes, cherries, and raisins

Hors d'oeuvres

The Healthy Substitutes

Bran crackers with or without fat-free cream cheese and jelly

Whole grain waffles, such as Van's

Rice cakes

Jell-O

Fruit ice pops, such as Crystal Light

Frozen chocolate mousse pops, those made by Weight Watchers, Yoplait, Tofutti, or the larger ones such as Skinny Cow and "Carb Control" by Klondike

Tootsie Roll pops

Sugar-free gum, preferably one that's not sweet (try Dentyne)

A chilled beverage, such as sugar-free lemonade or flavored mineral water

A creamy low-calorie beverage (for an ice cream substitute), such as Alba Shakes or Jeff's Diet Chocolate Soda

Light popcorn *only* in individual serving bags, such as Knight's or Weight Watchers

Crispbreads, such as GG Scandinavian brand, Wasa Light, or Bran-a-Crisp

Soups in individual servings (instant or frozen)

Sunflower seeds in *individual* snack bags

Raw green vegetables, such as string beans, celery, and fennel

Individual-size low-fat cheeses that have to be unwrapped before you can eat them, such as Mini-Bonbel Lights

up tensions that have no place to go. By the time he gets home, Jack is too tired to go to sleep and do much except watch TV. But Jack has never been able to sit in front of the tube without crunching on something. By the time he walked into my office, he weighed more than 300 pounds.

Jack wasn't particular about what he crunched. When I suggested to Jack that he toss out the junk snacks and substitute as many raw green beans as he wanted to eat, Jack's eyes lit up. As a health statistician, Jack knew full well that green beans are loaded with disease-fighting phytonutrients. Jack made the switch that night, and like many of my clients, he's now sailing along as a trim person snacking on raw vegetables.

Smart food strategy has the power to shift dangerous behavior in the direction of benign behavior. It liberated Jack and my other clients from the destructive cycle of "stress, eat, get fat." Smart food strategy removed the most painful part of the cycle: the negative consequence. Jack still crunches nonstop on string beans while he watches TV, but the consequence now is a positive one.

By overconsuming nonfattening vegetables instead of junk food, you're actually extending your life and reducing the risk factors for many serious diseases. Just making the switch from junk food to a health-giving food will give you a feeling of greater power over your life.

WHY WEIGHT LOSS IS BETTER THAN PROZAC

When it comes to mood elevation, I have found that all the chocolates of France, all the pizza of Italy, or all the ice cream of Häagen-Dazs will never elevate mood as much as losing weight, looking better, and feeling in control again. The most effective Prozac in the world is to take charge of your weight. I have a favorite mantra: "Happy or sad, rich or poor, it's still better being thin!" Even if you want to be miserable today, it's better to be thin and miserable than fat and miserable. Anyway you look at it, thin comes out ahead!

If eating could make people happy, then the heaviest people in the world would be the happiest. We all know that's not true, yet it's very easy to understand why we so often lose sight of it: There is massive confusion in our society between pleasure and happiness.

The heroin user, shooting that drug into her vein, has such feelings of pleasure that it overcomes the normal human revulsion to pain and needles. But that very pleasure destroys the possibility of happiness in a human life.

When you think about all the pain caused by the gaining and regaining of weight as a result of mood eating, you realize that "comfort foods" are a major cause of *discomfort* in human life. It's important that we realize that there are destructive pleasures—and that what we learned to be a benign comfort of our childhood may have become a destructive pleasure of our adulthood.

One of the most destructive aspects of mood eating goes almost totally unrecognized: Mood eating deceives us into living as mimics. When someone hurts or disappoints you, you then disappoint yourself by breaking with your weight program and gaining weight simply because you were eating over *their* behavior. It's rather ironic that when we eat because someone or something has made us angry or upset, we then also get angry with ourselves for doing it. It's a no-win pattern.

If you stop and reflect, most of the annoyances that prompt you to mood-eat—whether it's children's behavior or a comment made by a boss or relative—are not as important as the harm you do to your body and psyche by perpetuating a cycle of mood eating. By perpetuating this cycle, you perpetuate a sense of being unable to cope without dependence on food.

Many of my clients who faced terrible crises during the time they were working with me have told me that applying these new strategies that prevented them from turning to chocolates or peanuts became one of the greatest sources of strength in their lives. Whenever you use strategy, it puts you in control. Strategy empowers you to deal with the agenda of your life. You are no longer reacting as a victim but are the leader in your own life.

The Sixth Thin Commandment:

Take Control of
Your Favorite Foods

COMMANDMENT ESSENTIALS

- Limit frequency, availability, and quantity of your favorite
  foods.
- Make "I don't begin; I don't have any problem" your mantra.
- Save your calories for special meals, not everyday junk.
- Remember to think historically.
- Don't visit the dessert table for "just a look."

LET'S FACE IT: Many of your favorite foods are high in calories, and some of them may have gotten you into trouble in the
past. But that doesn't mean you can't still enjoy them.

With a smart game plan, you can eat your favorite foods
without having to wear them.

As so many of the winners at weight control have discovered,
the dual strategies of *Box It In* and *Box It Out* are powerful solutions
that make it easy to succeed at keeping high-calorie foods in your
life without gaining weight. You don't have to give up the treats
you love. *These techniques let you take control of your favorite foods, so
they don't take control of you.*

To *Box In* a food means you include it in your diet. The goal is always to keep as many favorite foods as possible in your life—and also to keep wearing your favorite size.

To *Box Out* means you exclude a food or type of food (such as bite-size snacks that are easy to pop into your mouth) from your diet. For some people, certain foods create such powerful cravings that they need to be treated separately. And although that may sound difficult, the majority of my clients have told me that among all the skills they've developed for managing their weight, Box It Out is the single most effective, easy-to-use way to maintain success at weight control.

Together, Box It In and Box It Out provide a set of tools that can free you forever from overeating your problem foods—and still let you enjoy them without gaining weight.

BOXING IN YOUR FAVORITE FOODS

Eating much-loved foods without putting on pounds is exactly what trips up so many people in their weight-control efforts. It may be the biggest stumbling block that you have faced over and over in the past. So, obviously, *this is one of the central issues of weight-control success.*

To stay trim and still eat what you love is a real skill—and an important mark of the winners at weight control. *The strategy that will allow you to master your favorite foods, once and for all, may be the most powerful tool you can take from this book.* For thousands of my clients, it's brought a permanent victory over their weight by controlling calories, limiting temptations, and ending their continual struggle with food.

Let's start by looking at the techniques that can help you to be thin for life, too.

1. **Limit frequency.** Enjoy your favorite food only at a specified time. Have it on designated days, or only in certain restaurants, or when served to you at a party. Whether you include it in your diet regularly or only on special occasions will depend on the food and your personal history with it.

2. **Limit availability.** Keep tempting foods out of your line of vision at home, and avoid eye contact with them in restaurants

and at other social events. One of the major triggers for wanting something is seeing it and smelling it. The studies on eating behavior are very clear about a simple fact: The more you see and are around the fattening foods you love, the more you will be tempted to eat them, the more you'll have cravings to battle, and the more you'll weigh. Being in control at home makes it easier to be in charge outside. If you're sloppy with your food consumption in private, it will have a ripple effect in public.

3. **Limit quantity.** Buy your favorite food in single serving sizes, serve it only in individual portions, and don't store it in large quantities.

Paula, a pediatrician with a fondness for desserts, allows herself to eat pies and cakes, but she lives by the rule that she will never buy a dessert for herself and bring it home. She can order it out or enjoy it when it's offered to her at the home of a friend, although she holds herself to no more than once a week.

She also allows herself to bake a sweet course when she's entertaining, but she prepares the dessert in individual portions so there are no extras to tempt her. If any is left over, she sends it home with someone else or quietly throws it out *before* the last guest leaves. Paula knows that by establishing how often she eats the food that she finds the most seductive and by reducing her opportunity to be around it, she can stay on track with her weight control—and her food control!

Another client, Cynthia, a travel agent, has a history of abusing Pepperidge Farm Milano cookies. But she's able to keep them in her life without danger by *never* buying a bag for her home. Instead, she keeps a bag in her office, in a closet far away from her desk, where it's not in her line of vision or easy to reach. At night, she takes home two cookies—no more, no less—and enjoys them after dinner.

I do the same as Cynthia with my evening dessert, which features a Van's 7-Grain Belgian waffle. When I kept a box at home, and I saw it every time I opened the freezer, I found I'd eat more waffles and continue to be tempted and think about them more often. I discovered, however, the perfect solution. I now keep a box in a freezer in my office, and each night I bring home a Belgian waffle. I make strawberry shortcake by topping the waffle with a few strawberries and some fat-free Reddi-wip. It's my favorite dessert, and I get to have it every night with no weight gain—and no tug of war with temptation!

Among recent findings from the National Weight Control Registry, in a survey of men and women who lost weight and kept it off, it was reported that two out of three of the "masters of weight control *keep problem foods out of their house and out of sight."* Like my clients, these winners at long-term weight control have discovered the value of Box It In techniques.

When you're aware that a certain food can sabotage you, that it can be a double-edged sword between pleasure and pain, you will be more likely to stay alert to not abusing it. The strategy of Boxing It In lets you stay on the side of pleasure, by keeping your attention on your problem food. This is a great psychological advantage because *those who stay focused, stay trim.*

When you follow the new rules you've established for yourself, you turn off your automatic pilot for eating and become more selective, wise, and careful in your food choices. Instead of randomly consuming at will, you can develop a personal strategy that will free you for the rest of your life from the snares that have repeatedly tripped you up. It's very empowering to set boundaries based on your own behavior, lifestyle, and history—and then to see the positive results in your life. When you consistently honor your new guidelines, you're sure to always be successful!

Eat and Be Merry

Many of my clients practice Boxing It In at holidays, family picnics, or other special events. They give themselves the pleasure of eating cake on their birthday or sampling every dish on the holiday table.

Weight gain over the holiday season doesn't come from one feast. The danger is in the foods and the trays of baked goods left out in the office and at home in the days before and after the holidays as well as the leftovers. The secret to getting through these events in your life is to Box In special meals on the holiday itself, or the evening before, rather than to randomly eat whatever you see, whenever you see it, throughout the season.

The Tale of a Southern Belle and the Pleasure of Pecan Pie

One of my clients, Suzanna, a homemaker and mother, is from Atlanta. She lives in Sun Valley, Idaho, now, but her tastes have stayed true to her roots. She loves Southern cooking.

When I first met her, she had many trigger foods. She got them all under control after a while, except for one: pecan pie. She was absolutely committed to staying in charge of her weight, and she did not want to resign herself to missing the enjoyment of this rich dessert, so she found a solution that uses the Box It In technique of eating a favorite food only at a specified time.

She allows herself to eat as much pecan pie as she wants at two dinners when she returns to visit her family four times a year. She doesn't bake it the rest of the year, buy it, or order it in restaurants. She has moments of wanting it, but they pass swiftly. She doesn't mind waiting for the pleasure of her favorite nutty confection—and she's added a new meaning to the phrase: "There's no place like home."

It's really great news for my clients to realize that they don't have to give up the great dinners that mark their birthdays or other special events. Enjoying a fine meal is part of the celebration of life and a wise and appropriate use of food.

Of course, it's still important to be prepared when facing a problem food. One of my clients, with a fondness for pies and cakes, has a creative plan that she follows on Thanksgiving. She enjoys every bite of the pumpkin pie filling, but leaves the crust behind. She's happy to do it, because it isn't the crust that makes the pie special. Every pie has a crust. It's the pumpkin filling that's her passion. With Box It In strategy, she can keep this favorite and unique taste in her life while avoiding the food that would sabotage her success at weight control.

Italian rum cake is a particular pleasure of mine, and I do some Boxing In with it. On Christmas day, I allow myself to eat as many slices as I want, knowing I won't be seeing rum cake again soon. Although I don't limit the quantity that I eat on this one day, I do limit the availability. This high-calorie treat won't be on my grocery list or appearing in my day-to-day life in the coming months, and that knowledge allows me to give myself the freedom for a delicious, special indulgence.

BOX IT IN OR OUT?

Maybe the food you love is pretzels or ice cream or brownies. Whatever it is, if you want it to remain in your life, you must take a good look at how, where, and when it is least likely to be a problem for you. *Your lifelong success at weight control depends on how well you handle the foods that tempt you the most.*

All of us want to keep all the foods we love in our life, all of the time. But that is just not realistic in an adult world. When we grow up, we accept that we can't have everything we want. We recognize the need to set priorities and be selective.

Selectivity is a part of living at peace with ourselves, and personal happiness is living out the vision that we have for our lives. If your vision is to see yourself as a trim person for all the years to come, then you will know that your favorite size has to come before your favorite food. You'll understand that what is essential for happiness is not the same as what is simply nice to have or "what looks interesting."

Since you can't have it all, all the time, your guidelines need to be: How much can you have? Where and when? And what food management style works best for you? What choices will help you to be "foodSmart?"—to spend your calories wisely?

With strategy, you can enjoy your favorite foods without putting on pounds. However, it works only if the food is indeed manageable. In certain cases, there may be a few or perhaps just one or two foods that can't be handled in this way because they trigger such powerful cravings in people with physiological hypersensitivities.

But the good news, the promise of the Box It In strategy is this: *Anything that you love that you can truly control can be a part of your life forever.*

Use these three key techniques to guide you:

1. If you can have "just a sliver" when it's served to you, but you would overeat it if you were in your home, then *only* eat it when you're a guest in someone's home or *only* in restaurants.

And limit those occasions, too, to special events, or hold yourself to eating it in specified restaurants.

2. If you can Box In a food at home, be sure to keep it under "wraps." Cover tempting leftovers with aluminum foil—not in see-through plastic. Store them out of sight in the farthest reaches of the refrigerator, even hidden in the vegetable compartment. Keep other snacks and treats in closed cabinets, the more remote and inconvenient the better.

3. If you eat it compulsively when it's in the house, then *never* bring it home. If you buy it for yourself, limit the amount by choosing small packages and single-serving sizes—or throw out the extras in the package before you put it in your kitchen.

As I've suggested before, there may be a few foods for some of us that are not a good choice for Boxing In. They ignite such strong desires, they activate my F-Q principle—first you have a little, then the *frequency* increases, and eventually, invariably, an increase in *quantity* follows. These foods trigger *ongoing cravings* and *obsessive thoughts* and lead you into a process that wears down your motivation to stay in charge. It's the pattern that you must break if you're going to be a lifelong winner at weight control.

As you consider your problem foods, you may conclude that it might be easier to Box Out one or two foods from your life. This is a critical choice, upon which your success hinges. *When you think historically and see that you have a long history of abuse with a certain food, that every time you've gone back to it, it's created powerful cravings and obsessive thoughts, and your weight has returned, then the key to control is realizing that the risk of eating it is not worth the momentary pleasure it may give.* It's far better to get a few foods out of your life—and still enjoy the figure that you want for life.

But how do you give up your favorite foods? Is it possible? Does it mean living with suffering, constant feelings of cravings and deprivation—feeling you're missing out on the fun? For most of my clients, the opposite has been true. They tell me repeatedly that their decision to Box Out a food has made their lives easier and their success at weight control far more certain. With the Box It

Out techniques that follow, you'll discover how this wonderful outcome can be yours too.

As always, you must be truthful with yourself. As Henry David Thoreau observed: *It takes two to speak the truth—one to speak it, another to hear it.* Through the pages of this book, I'm sharing the truths I've learned, but you must be honest with yourself about how they apply to your life. Otherwise you'll be "boxing yourself in" for a lifetime of weight problems.

Taking Control of a Food That Doesn't Work for You

For some people, when it comes to trigger foods, good intentions just aren't enough. You can know that Box It In is *not working* for you if any of these statements describe you:

- You think about a food more and more often even though you may be eating it regularly.
- Your cravings return or increase.
- You continually renegotiate the terms of the agreement you made with yourself so you can eat the food more often.
- When you stop or limit the food, you lose weight.
- When you return to eating it, you start gaining weight back.
- You break promises to yourself about how much or how often you'll consume it.

If you recognize these symptoms, don't kid yourself. Talking about "just a little" or "just this once" is the road back to fat. In such a situation, it's time to admit that a food doesn't work for you. It's time to Box It Out of your life.

It's important to understand that there is a considerable difference between doing without something of our own accord and being made to do without it. With this strategy, it is *not* that you *can't have* your favorite food or that anyone is taking it away from you, but that you are being honest with yourself. You are choosing to free yourself from weight problems, cravings, and constant battles that wear you down. In a world full of life-threatening illness, starvation, and homelessness, one food or type of food is never *really* a necessity—but it may be necessary to get it out of your life so you can have the life you want. Never lose your good values; most of the people living on this planet today have never spent a millisecond of their lives thinking about the food you think you can't live without.

One of the saddest lessons in my practice is that I've seen thousands of clients whose journey through a continuing series of weight failures mirrors the similar struggle of millions of Americans—people who have never succeeded on a weight program because of just one or two foods. I've worked with many clients who were heavy in their 60s because of the very same foods that made them heavy in their 30s, 40s, and 50s. How painful to realize that they would never have known one dieting failure after another had they simply Boxed Out one or two foods. They have spent decades being heavy—along with the physical and emotional costs—because of these foods! And one of the laments I hear most frequently in the clients who have successfully Boxed Out a food is: "Why didn't I realize this sooner?"

In choosing to avoid a certain food, you are freeing yourself from constant weight problems, cravings, and the unending battle with temptations that wear down your willpower.

This is what John Drybread had in mind when he wrote: *For those who are given to excess, abstinence is easier than moderation.*

Once a food is eliminated from your diet, you will be able to live with a new sense of freedom and control—and most of all success. My clients who have made a decision to Box Out a food have discovered one of the great secrets of weight control: *Far from feeling deprived without a certain food, they felt liberated—from cravings and old struggles and from years of failure with their weight—and they find it's much easier to live without it.*

At one time, I made the mistake of thinking, perhaps as you may think, that it would be *harder* to eliminate a food than to eat it in moderation. But my clients' successes taught me that the opposite is true—*it's easier!*

Some of my clients, when they reached the maintenance level in their diets, would respond to my suggestion that they go back to a certain food with a horrified expression and an adamant "No! Never!"

In making this adjustment, it's critical that you know how to outmaneuver your psyche's deprivation mechanism. Never say

"You can't have it." It's not true, and it may trigger feelings of deprivation. Say to yourself instead, "It doesn't work for me." This way you don't fall into the "Eve Complex" of something becoming more attractive because it's forbidden. You can have all you want, whenever you want. But if you do, you will never have the life or the control that you want. You are using your "life smarts" and freely choosing not to have it so you can choose to be trim.

"I don't miss it. It's easier if I don't begin," they'd tell me again and again. "It might reactivate my cravings. I'm afraid to go back." Statements of this kind helped me understand how powerful it can be for some people to *not take a taste* of a food.

The same message kept coming back to me, and the lesson was clear: *To Box Out a food is one of the most powerful and surprisingly easy techniques for mastering cravings.*

My clients follow the same rule for high-carbohydrate items, such as pasta. Or they Box In the quantity of the food by ordering it as an appetizer, a small serving size. And they always have pomodoro sauce (tomatoes without oil).

In this way, they've been able to sample all the magnificent creations of the great chefs of the world—and emerge unscathed!

Instead of food items, they buy themselves beautiful clothes or other special souvenirs.

At hotels, they don't take the key for the wet bar, and they request no turndown service, since many hotels leave candy or cookies on the pillow at night. If there's a welcome basket full of goodies when they arrive, they ask the bellman to remove it.

Save your calories for special meals, not everyday junk!

As I discuss in the Third Thin Commandment, The Problem May Be in the Food, Not in You, the reason you've been unable to moderate a food may have little or nothing to do with your willpower or strength of character. Certain foods trigger your appetite and overpower the appetite control center in the brain. It may have to do with your own biological hypersensitivity to the taste, look, or aroma of a certain food.

When a food is a part of life, it enhances life, but when it becomes the centerpiece of a human life—when it comes before your appearance and your control over your own body and subjects you to continuing failure at something that is so precious to your happiness and health, when it comes before your wardrobe, self-image, and promises that you make to yourself—then that food does not enhance your life, but diminishes it! Eating such a food does not free you; it imprisons you—and sentences you to a lifelong struggle with your weight and with failure.

This is the change in thinking that is so important to understand: Eating the food *is* the deprivation because it deprives you of reaching your critical life goals. And when you make this shift in your mind, you truly come to see a great new truth in a new light: *Boxing Out a food is not about deprivation, but about liberation.*

The prevailing thinking in the professional diet field says we should give in and indulge cravings occasionally because too much deprivation sabotages weight loss, leads to bingeing, and wears down resolve. You may have read many times that if you feel deprived, your diet will fail, but that's only half of the truth.

It's correct *if* you don't change your thinking. But it's *not true* when you realize that just one or two foods have stolen your figure, your favorite wardrobe, and your success at managing your weight. It's not true when you understand that by *not* eating a certain food, you will actually be deactivating the craving mechanism within your brain and your psyche. You'll be turning off cravings forever. When you learn to say "No, thank you," to a food *and* use the techniques of Box It Out, you'll discover, as so many of my clients have, that you will be saying "yes" to being thin for life.

In her books *Thin for Life* and *Eating Thin for Life,* author Anne M. Fletcher, M.S., R.D., the noted nutritionist, studied 208 weight-loss masters who had lost at least 20 pounds and kept them off for 3 or more years. She found that *more than half* of these people just avoid the foods they know will trigger overeating. Obviously these winners know that beginning with a little will lead to more and that *not even starting is the smart way to go.*

If a problem food has been in your life for years, if you've struggled with your weight every time you've tried to eat it in moderation, then you have the evidence that if you continue consuming it in the same way, you will never achieve success at weight control. As I've said before, the mark of smart people is that they avoid doing, again and again, what doesn't work.

GETTING RID OF A FOOD THAT'S SABOTAGED YOU, AGAIN AND AGAIN

What do you do about the chocolate chip cookies, nibble foods, breadbaskets, or other foods that always seem to be getting the better of you? Follow these guidelines for Boxing Out troublesome foods.

1. **Shift your thinking.** Living trim doesn't mean you have to give up the pleasure of fine dining or even most of your favorite foods. By making a conscious choice to avoid one food or type of food, you know that you *can* eat it any time you want, but if you do, you would be *depriving yourself* of a lifetime of being thin, in control, and free of cravings. Realize, also, that not eating this food will free up thousands or tens of thousands of calories per month to enjoy other foods you love.

2. **Set a date when you are going to stop eating it, and reward yourself for the decision.** Buy yourself a present, such as a new outfit in a smaller size. Tell yourself you can have the food again, from a certain age on, such as 75.

3. **Tell yourself: It's not an option.** The human psyche is prone to negotiate boundaries where pleasure is involved, but when it hears an unequivocal "No!" it becomes surprisingly obedient and respects the line.

4. **Remember to think historically.** Calorie counters say, "What's wrong with a taste?" My clients and I know that's a big mistake. Taste buds don't care if they get a little bite or many big bites—once they're reactivated, they're back in control. After that, eating your trigger food is like throwing gas on a fire. One taste can reactivate the craving memory of a lifetime. It's not about the calories but the cravings! Once you're struggling with cravings, weight control feels much harder. The size of the portion is irrelevant to the power of the cravings that will follow.

5. **Avoid eye contact.** No one ever graduated from baking school for turning out ugly looking cookies, cakes, and tarts. *No eye contact allowed* is a smart strategy.

6. **Don't allow thinking that sabotages you.** Don't tolerate an inner voice that speaks to you about your problem food.

Avoid reading about it in recipes, magazines, and restaurant reviews.

7. **Give up resentments and thinking "It's not fair."** Wayne W. Dyer, Ph.D, a leading therapist and bestselling author, counsels that when you are filled with resentments, you turn over control of your emotional life. But when you depersonalize an issue, you have no need to feel resentment, and you "immunize" yourself against negativity and doubt. Remember: The problem may be in the food, not in you, so it doesn't work for you—unless you want to wear it!

8. **Cut off food curiosity.** If you've given up desserts, there's no reason to visit a dessert table for "just a look." If pasta is a problem for you, don't study the spaghetti and ravioli selections in a restaurant menu. You have no reason to give your problem food any role in your life.

9. **Make a public announcement about your food choices.** If you tell everyone at a party or at your table that you don't eat a certain food, you commit yourself to not eating it. The power of embarrassment is greater than willpower.

10. **Try not to buy it for your home or buy a substitute.** If you must buy it for other family members, select a small supply in single serving sizes. Or purchase a variety of the food that appeals to you the least. If you like Cherry Garcia ice cream, buy another flavor for the family that doesn't tempt you. (Not keeping it in your immediate environment permanently is the most helpful strategy of all. That's what the winners strive to do.)

11. **Reinforce your commitment with the single most powerful statement that supports your resolve: I don't begin; I don't have any problem.** This is what almost all of my clients say when they see their Boxed Out food. It cuts off thinking and debating. For some, I have qualified the phrase: *If I don't take the first little taste, I don't begin. I don't have a problem,* since I found that the negotiators among us could often get into trouble by saying to themselves, *I won't begin, but I'll just have a little taste.* But, of course, having a little taste is indeed beginning. As I have noted, *the size of the portion is irrelevant to the power of the crav-*

ings that will follow—not to mention the reawakening of the interest in and the thinking about the food again.

12. **Reward yourself.** Replace the "food treat" psychology of your childhood with the adult reward system of a new outfit, vacation, or something special you want. You deserve rewards, and being trim will be one of them.

You may think that it's endlessly difficult to refuse a food you've always loved, but with smart strategy, the once seemingly impossible becomes possible—even easy. The truth is that cravings fade over time if they're not reinforced through tasting and other visual cues. And once you make a decision to give up a food because it doesn't work for you, life becomes simpler. When you've made a clear choice, within a short time, your psyche will accept the change, and you'll stop thinking about the food that once occupied so much of your thoughts.

Dean Ornish, M.D., the director of the Preventive Medicine Research Institute and the author of four bestselling books about diet and health, has come to a similar conclusion. *Despite conventional wisdom, he writes, it is actually easier to make big changes in diet all at once than to make small, gradual ones . . . Most people find that they feel so much better so quickly that the choices become clearer and worth making . . . to increase the joy of living.*

When You Can't Remove a Food from Sight

Many people find that they can say "no" to a food for a short time, but if they sit with it, whether it's a breadbasket or a tray of cookies, it soon starts to wear down their resolve.

My client, Matthew, an entertainment lawyer, frequently dines out with clients. Since he can't avoid eye contact with the breadbasket, his Boxed Out food, he uses the clever strategy of announcing at the beginning of the meal that the rolls look delicious, but he's sworn off them.

"It works every time," he tells me. "Once I've identified myself as a non-bread eater, I know I'll be embarrassed if I contradict myself. So I'm not tempted."

SUBSTITUTION IS OFTEN THE KEY TO SUCCESS

My client, Annette, remains untroubled when buying cakes and cookies for her husband and children, although she has Boxed Out

What to Do When You're Falling Out of Control

Even the most successful weight strategist can hit a rough patch sometime. If you find yourself suddenly falling into constantly overeating, your control is slipping, and you may even be bingeing, these crisis-intervention techniques may help stop your slide:

1. **Remember the lesson of The Fourth Thin Commandment, "Structure Gives Control."** Immediately write out an eating plan for the next 24 hours, several days, a week, or longer. The further you can plan ahead, the more the strategy can help put you back in charge.

2. **Make it easy to do the right thing.** Remove from your home any foods that are a temptation for you. Watch out for products that might not have been a problem before but may now have a new appeal.

3. **Don't turn a detour into a catastrophe.** Turn off the thinking that suggests that because you've gone overboard, you're out of control and you might as well continue overeating.

4. **Fight the temptation to eat too little.** Many people, when they feel they've consumed too many calories in one day, will go too far in the other direction for the next day or two. They'll undereat, which leaves them hungry and more prone to losing control. Avoid this common mistake by eating healthy meals and snacks every 3 to 4 hours throughout the day.

5. **If you've gone back to a trigger food, especially sweets and/or a flour-and-sugar product, and you've reactivated cravings and recurring thoughts about it, you can address the problem by "throwing protein at it."** This tactic isn't well supported in current diet thinking, but I've found that a diet, for a day or two, that consists of as many as four to five small meals that contain a good source of low-fat protein will stabilize blood-sugar levels and reduce strong cravings as well as any increased appetite. If you've been eating too much creamy ice cream, for in-

products made with white flour, fat, and sugar. She shrewdly chooses varieties made with raisins and nuts, which have no appeal for her. Another client buys pastries filled with whipped cream, which she dislikes, for her family. These women know how to strategize!

stance, the substitute of a creamy, cold dilled egg salad (see my recipe on page 221) may jump-start you back on track with a healthy eating plan. I'm not suggesting this as an everyday technique, but as a strategy to turn to when you're feeling especially vulnerable. You might even overeat protein a bit to be sure your blood-sugar levels remain even.

6. **If you're continuing to crave sugar, try saturating your taste buds with salty, spicy, or hot food.** Pickles, salsas, and other hot sauces may reduce your cravings. You might also try a sugar substitute in liquid form, which most people are less likely to abuse, such as diet sodas, or a diet shake such as the Alba Shake, or my Jeff's Diet Chocolate or Vanilla sodas.

7. **If you've been overindulging in salty foods, such as pretzels, nuts, or chips, try pickles to knock out your cravings or my "fried" zucchini sticks or chips** (see my recipe on page 219).

8. **Sometimes eating isn't about food. You may be upset, angry, or hurt. Talk it over with a friend or counselor, or keep a journal.** Once you express your feelings in speech or writing, they're out, and they become easier to manage in appropriate ways. By simply venting emotions, you increase the likelihood of immediately returning to control.

Your situation might also be the result of a change in your attitude. Perhaps you're pleased with what you weigh, you may have recently dropped a number of pounds, and you've lost some of your motivation to be careful with your diet. In such a case, it's important to make a decision that you won't allow yourself to become sloppy with your eating habits.

Remember the advice I've given you to *get the mood out of the food*. Take back your power. Don't allow other people or external events to control what you put into your body. Refuse to eat a single extra calorie because of the negative people who may be in your life.

Remember my client Joan? Once she started to eat cookies, she couldn't stop, but she had no trouble with chocolate mousse parfait. Other clients who can't eat cookies have discovered they can have a single Van's whole grain waffle or two Aunt Jemima Light Pancakes for dessert at home. Both these products are flaky and cakelike and can satisfy a sweet craving for about 100 calories.

In my diet section (see page 294), I'll give you a list of the best-tasting substitutes available in America today that will supply all the rich tastes and the great looks that make foods so tempting, but without the calories that make them fattening.

THE MORE YOU EAT, THE MORE YOU CRAVE

If you're hypersensitive to food containing sugar, flour, crunch, or fat, having a little of it doesn't help, and it may hurt. As I've discussed, these ingredients as well as some others can actually overpower the appetite control center and change the brain's neurochemistry. You can come to constantly crave sweet baked goods or other products to the exclusion of alternative foods.

But if you cut out these foods and use the strategies to Box It Out, the cravings will begin to weaken and eventually go away. And there's more great news: One of the major findings of my work is that when you eliminate the handful of foods that tempt you the most, your appetite for all foods seems to fall significantly as well as your interest in them. It may be due to cutting back on the level of carbohydrates or simply diminishing temptation, but whatever the mechanism, you have much less hunger- and food-obsessed thinking and much greater success with your weight control. The majority of my clients have discovered that they no longer crave or think about their former problem food, and they're only tempted by it if they happen to see or be seated near it for some length of time. Even then, the craving is no longer an overwhelming compulsion, but just a mild feeling.

DON'T FORGET TO REWARD YOURSELF

Another characteristic of the human psyche, one of the strongest, is that it likes to be given special acknowledgment with treats and presents. I encourage my clients to celebrate their success with weight control by indulging in any luxury that would make them happy.

I also tell them that now that they've grown up, they need to choose adult gifts for themselves. Children are rewarded with a cookie, a grown-up deserves presents that enhance life much more significantly.

When you're pleased with yourself and proud of how you look, a trip to a tropical paradise or just a visit to the local beach or community pool can give you a chance to look great in shorts or your bathing suit. It can do wonders for your self-esteem. It's especially satisfying to buy new clothing in your favorite size, and the pleasure strengthens your commitment to continue following The Thin Commandments, which are your ticket to a lifetime of being trim.

One of my clients, an executive at a financial management company, understood the power that the right purchase could harness for keeping up his motivation. He bought himself a Ferrari. "Even if I bought myself the most expensive suit I could find, I still might let myself slip and gain back some weight," he explained to me. "But I know I'll never let myself become so fat again that I couldn't fit into my great car. It was worth every penny because it guarantees that I will always be thin. Every time I drive it, I'm reminded of how much I want to live this life that I have worked so hard to earn."

Box It In and Box It Out can bring success to you, too. With these powerful strategies, you and you alone decide what foods you can and cannot control. You choose the foods that you will abstain from, limit, or continue to eat when you like based on your food history, sensitivities, and preferences. When you're in charge, when you have a vision of yourself as a trim person, when you know what is important to you, and you set the boundaries that work to help you reach your goals, you become a winner at weight control. You gain freedom forever from food struggles—and a lifelong assurance of living thin.

The Seventh Thin Commandment:

Slips Should Teach You, Not Defeat You

COMMANDMENT ESSENTIALS

- Error control is the essence of weight control.
- Don't say "I blew it" if you make an eating mistake.
- Don't undereat in an attempt to compensate for cheating the previous day.
- Discover your predictable pattern in eating mistakes.
- Use binge-busters to end a craving.
- Don't go hungry.
- Find something to do, such as reading a book or knitting, to help get your mind off your craving.
- Think substitution, not deprivation.
- Put a negative association with the foods that tempt you most.

WOULDN'T IT BE GREAT IF THERE were just one thing that made you a winner at weight control? There is.

One characteristic marks every winner I've worked with and eludes everyone who doesn't succeed: Those who master weight control learn from their mistakes instead of losing to them.

You may think that winners make fewer mistakes, that they're a different breed of human. The truth is they're not. They're just like you. They make mistakes. *It's how they deal with their mistakes* that makes them winners. They treat a diet slip like any human error. They cut it off, see what went wrong, and take steps to prevent it from happening again. *Winners deal with mistakes by learning from them; failures deal with mistakes by blindly repeating them!*

Errors can slow your progress and weaken your focus. *Our goal is to prevent error, not promote it.* However, this book is designed to meet the needs of how real people behave in the real world as opposed to a perfect one. Human beings make mistakes. "To err is human."

But did you ever think you could make mistakes and *still lose weight*—in fact, lose all the weight you want? With the right skills, you can. Very few of my clients have perfect weeks, but almost all of them lose weight!

You will make mistakes—this is certain. But equally certain is that *these errors do not have to lead to weight gain, but in fact can lead to you being a master at stopping them quickly and keeping them at bay in the future. There can be no success at weight control without successful error control!*

Past mistakes do *not* mean future failure.

Charles was a successful New York architect but had failed on so many diets that he didn't think I could help much. "How long have you been trying?" I asked.

"Thirty-plus years," he said. "Just like my parents, a new diet every couple of months. I guess it's in my genes."

Maybe there's something of Charles in some of you, readers. You've tried many times over the years to lose weight and just as many times not succeeded. Maybe you, too, had heavy parents and feel genetics can't be overcome. The good news is that none of these suspicions is true, and the fact that you are reading this proves that you somehow suspect this!

THE SINGLE BIGGEST MISTAKE

I told Charles that just the fact that he came to me proved that he still believed he could win the game of weight control. "I always believe at first," he said, "but then something happens, and I blow the whole thing. I don't really see what you can do to stop that."

I told him he was right about one thing: I couldn't stop him from sooner or later making an error on his diet, because everyone makes mistakes! "In fact," I said, "I'm sure I make more mistakes than many of my clients! But what I can help you with is *how you learn from your mistakes.* That's what will make the difference this time! There's just one mistake you have to promise you'll never make again."

"Which one?" he asked.

"Just promise me—and more important, promise yourself—*that you'll never again say, 'I blew it.'*"

He looked shocked. "Just never say, 'I blew it'?"

"Or any of its familiar variants: 'I blew the day. The day is ruined. It's all over.' That's the only real mistake that leads to failure in weight control. Everything else will be your learning laboratory."

He smiled and said, "It's a deal."

That deal helped Charles lose 65 pounds over the following months!

A few years later, I saw his picture in the newspaper, still looking very trim, at the dedication of a building he designed in mid-Manhattan. I called him to congratulate him. We talked a bit and then he said, "You know, Doctor, I still have never made that great mistake!"

I paused because it had been awhile—I wasn't sure what mistake he meant.

"The single biggest mistake!" he quickly filled me in. "Ever since the first time we met in your office, I never once have said, 'I blew the day'!"

THE BIGGEST CAUSE OF EXCESS POUNDS IS *NOT* A FOOD

It's not even a behavior—it's a *mindset.* It's a mental habit that reacts to a diet slip by giving up, "letting the screen go blank." When dieters cheat (eat a high-calorie dessert, say), this one error tends to become a reason to stop *all* their efforts at weight control. Instead of handling it like any human error—asking, "What can I learn from this?"—they say, "Well, I blew it, I might as well blow the rest of the day (or the weekend, or longer)."

This "I blew it" syndrome is different from the momentary *feeling* of "I blew it," which we all may get after eating too much. Winners certainly have had this *feeling* about a particular meal or food. But then they become more careful and balance the excess with smart eating. *The failures say, "I blew it," and let their mental screens go blank. Their eating gets careless, and this carelessness engulfs the day and often the next day(s). This is the "I blew it" syndrome.* Something in you says that you might as well eat all you can for the rest of the day so you can *"get it all in" before going back on your diet. I also call this "the last meal syndrome"* and tell my clients: "It will never be your last meal. You're not being thrown in the dungeon. There will be too much food in your life, never too little. So don't act as if a great famine is about to start." The good news, though, is that these mistakes can easily be contained, using the techniques in this book.

One of the great lessons in my work is how many people approach weight control with the idea "I'll either be perfect or perfectly horrible." They don't think this way when they learn any other skill, such as knitting, using their software, or even parenting.

Of course, the motive for weight loss is often so strong that most people *do* start a weight program perfectly. They're in what I call the "weight-loss zone," just to see the numbers come down. This is why people can give up food entirely and start out with just liquid protein drinks. When you're miserable because you don't fit into your clothes, doing any diet brings relief, even if you feel that you're swimming underwater, holding your breath to do it perfectly. But as the pounds come off, and the clothes get loose, and the compliments start, experience has shown that sooner or later you'll have to come up for "error."

And when you do make a mistake—as we all do—*don't continue and make the fatal mistake of saying, "I blew the day."* Because this syndrome is *the* dividing line between those who lose weight only to gain it back and those who keep it off forever!

Why the "I Blew It" Syndrome Is Terminal to Diets

No one ever gets heavy from one mistake, one meal of extra calories, a bag of candies, or even several hors d'oeuvres at a cocktail party! It's only when you lose control of the eating that comes after the mistake that the weight gain begins.

The "I blew it" syndrome . . .

- Sets up an impossible tension in your life: that you have to be either perfect or a failure
- Lets your mental screen go blank, so you shut down everything that you've learned about food management
- Lets mistakes pile up, which drowns your motivation, skews your perspective, and overwhelms your willpower
- Destroys focus on your eating and weight control. (Studies all show that staying *focused* on your eating behavior is what makes you a winner.)
- Is self-defeating. It cuts off learning from the mistake and locks you into a pattern of repeating it
- Only helps you learn that you're gaining weight, which is obvious
- Ruins your chance to cut off the mistake and keep any weight gain small and temporary
- Keeps you from proving to yourself that you *can* stop and correct the error, a tremendous source of empowerment
- Turns a few minutes of unwise eating into something that will take days, months, or even years to make up for. It's not time efficient
- Paralyzes you into a mode of helplessness that lets one mistake end up becoming thousands of calories
- Doesn't do justice to your intelligence, your life smarts
- Doesn't make you lose weight; it only makes you lose hope. Cutting off the error does the opposite: It builds hope and gives you power
- Doesn't answer the most important question of all: *What went wrong in this situation, and what could I do differently?*

ERROR CONTROL IS THE ESSENCE OF WEIGHT CONTROL

Erica was a struggling actress who was "tired of playing the fat jolly friend of the romantic lead." She apologized for crying, but she felt that she was wasting the years of her youth with failure after failure in weight control. I handed her a box of tissues and said, "Erica, those years were anything but wasted. There are patterns and reasons why you've failed, and from those lessons, you can script a new future. That experience can show you just what you need to do to get the weight you want."

She wiped her eyes and sighed. "It just seems no matter how hard I try, ice cream defeats me!" I had to laugh, and she smiled. "Erica, food has no IQ. It has no life smarts."

"Maybe not, but there's something in me that has to have Rocky Road!"

"Do you really think your eating mistakes result from demonic possession?"

She burst out laughing and said, "Well I did grow up in the Dakota!" (The Dakota is the New York City building where they filmed the movie *Rosemary's Baby*.) Then she sighed again and said, "I just feel like a complete failure."

"If food is winning against us, it doesn't mean we're weak, pathetic souls beyond redemption. It just means we have to figure out a better strategy. Most people who get into trouble with weight control haven't really failed, they've failed to plan. Error control is the basis of that plan. You've just never had a strategy for error control. You're certainly not a complete failure!"

Erica's beautiful eyes had turned serious. "I never thought of that before," she commented.

"Error control is one of the most neglected areas in my field, but I've found it to be the essence of weight control. Think about it. What weight-control program is known for its strong emphasis on error-control techniques?"

"None that I've heard of," she said. "This makes so much sense to me!"

Erica was one of my clients who realized from the start that this particular thin commandment was the ultimate shortcut! The phrase "I blew it" would never cross her lips. You could see her determination when she talked about a slip she made, eager to learn all she could from it!

Because she made this commandment her number one priority, Erica reached her desired weight as fast as any client I've ever had in her weight-control category. Error control is the essence of weight control. Letting your slips teach you and not defeat you goes to the heart of the weight problem. This commandment cuts across all the others because in following any of them (just like the real

10 Commandments), people make mistakes. So knowing how to control and learn from mistakes makes any commandment work more powerfully.

The Magic Bullet for Error Control

The first thing to do after making a mistake is to stop it as soon as you can. Contain the mistake before it turns into an overwhelming series of mistakes. Just as there are chain smokers, there are "chain eaters." Don't allow the chain to start, and you will succeed in weight control!

As soon as you finish eating the improper food or conclude the overeating episode, talk to yourself in a new way. *Instead of saying, "I blew it," say, "Stop now."* This breaks the "I blew it" syndrome instead of allowing you to keep eating as if your diet had just been proven useless. It hasn't at all! The overwhelming majority of my clients who have made one or two errors during the week but cut them off quickly still lost weight. If you stop the mistake before it turns into a chain, you can still lose some weight for the week and never gain it back!

That's why it's so important to change your self-talk after an eating mistake. You have to change your thinking in order to change your weight permanently! Instead of telling yourself, "I blew it," remember that failure (or even weight gain) doesn't come from one mistake but from "letting your screen go blank" and letting a 1-minute mistake multiply into a calorie mountain that crushes your diet. Tell yourself "Stop now," and don't start chain-eating, the deadliest threat to a diet I've found in all my years of work.

The longer you persist in your eating mistake—the more chain-eating you do—the harder it will be to get back on track. And by then you're making other mistakes, and you feel like you're just sinking deeper and deeper. So it's immensely important to have a strategy to contain the mistake before it turns into chain-eating.

THE 24-HOUR SECRET

In the course of helping thousands of people in their struggle not to chain-eat, one day it struck me that they all had something in common, a tendency not shown by winners: Most people who make a diet mistake will continue the pattern for the rest of the day! *I call it the "slip to sleep" syndrome.*

So know the following, and you can take steps to avoid it: If you cheat on your diet, you will be strongly tempted to cheat more and more for the rest of the day and often for the next 24 hours. If you make a conscious, focused effort not to fall into the pattern for the rest of the day and into the next, the temptation to cheat passes. With good strategy, you can immediately cut it off! You can get through this manageable period of time and make the cheating an isolated event. You end the cycle of bingeing from day to day, avert chain-eating, and do not gain weight from your slips. And that is the 24-Hour Secret.

From Slip to Sleep: The Critical Period

The essence of weight control is error control, and *the essence of error control is managing the period from slip to sleep.* If you have success in this short but crucial period, you will have success in getting to your optimal weight. In a very real sense, being a winner at weight control all boils down to this section, these words you are reading right now.

You're especially vulnerable from the time of your error to the time you go to bed. Most people tend to blow off the rest of the day, and often this spills into the next. *The battle of weight gain is won or lost in this critical period.*

Here's the core strategy my clients have found works best during this time.

• **Write out what you will eat for the rest of the day, meals as well as snacks.** This is the most successful strategy. Push yourself; force yourself to make this menu. Remember the Nike commercial, and "Just do it." Rally your energy for this one small step, and make a giant leap toward mastering your error. Take care to pick healthy foods you like, so you won't end up feeling deprived.

• **Write out tomorrow's menu as well.** And make sure the right foods will be available.

• **Do a brief mental rehearsal.** This technique—which I explain at the end of this chapter (see page 119)—will desensitize you to the power of any tempting food *before* you even encounter it.

• **Use diversion.** Plan some interesting activity for the rest of the day. Anything that occupies the mind will quickly divert it from thoughts about food and cravings. *Avoid boredom at all costs!* When you're bored, the thought of food seems extra interesting—not because you're hungry but just because it might "fill up" the empty time. The diversion may be as simple as making a few telephone calls or just staying busy with personal projects.

• **Commit to the menu you've written, from that point until you go to bed.** It's only a matter of hours. Anyone can comply.

Dealing with the "Day–After" Syndrome

The day after a slip is easier, but it still has dangers. First: *Be aware when you wake up that there is such a thing as the "Day-After Syndrome" so you'll be prepared.* You may find a heightened interest in your cheat food because the memory of its taste is still vivid. Your taste-bud memory has been strongly reinforced—particularly if your error food was a simple carbohydrate such as sugar or a white-flour product. Tell yourself: *It's not an option.* But also tell yourself that your interest in these foods will decline over the course of the day as your blood sugar evens out. You won't crave them forever, just a few more hours.

Here's the best strategy for the "Day-After Syndrome":

Start the day with exercise. Do *any* kind of exercise, even if it's for only 15 minutes. It's not just about burning calories; it's about *a healthy mindset.* It gives structure to your day, starts it with a positive commitment, and sets your mental focus to be careful and good to your body all day.

Go over your menu for the day. Make sure it's written out in advance and includes snacks and meals. *Pick only foods you like so you won't feel deprived!* The "day after" is not a good time to trigger that other PMS—the "Poor Me Syndrome." Choose foods you like, even if they have more calories, so a feeling of deprivation won't tempt you to repeat the errors of yesterday.

Don't undereat! This should be your most important goal today. *Do not attempt to undereat to compensate for yesterday.* This can end up making you too hungry on a day when the cravings may already be stronger than usual. *It's not about losing weight the next day; it's about not losing ground.* The key is rebuilding control and stopping the error pattern. Even if your scale may be up a few pounds—

don't panic. Probably most of this gain is water retention from salt and carbohydrate intake and will be gone tomorrow with proper eating. Avoid the scale entirely if it will cause too much negativity. And don't try to "catch up" with your weight loss in just 1 day—the day after.

Have a fourth meal. A fourth meal of low-calorie, low-fat protein keeps blood sugar at an optimal level. Stabilized blood sugar puts off your hunger and significantly reduces cravings. Schedule it on your menu for when you're most vulnerable (late afternoon for most people).

Use visualization. See yourself eating the proper meals and snacks you've written on your menu. And try this ultimate visualization: Put an article of clothing you love but is still too tight to wear where you'll see it during the day.

Reduce temptation. Don't go to restaurants you know are danger zones, and avoid food shopping if you can. Get rid of any leftovers or give them away. And try not to look at foods that aren't on your menu.

Reach out and keep busy. Catch up on overdue phone calls to upbeat people you like. The goal here is the same as from slip to sleep: Do something enjoyable to kill boredom and *block* food thoughts. If you don't want to talk to someone, try an enjoyable activity instead. Reaching out redirects the mind to one of the most interesting, fulfilling acts—connecting with another person you care about or a rewarding activity, *not* food.

I have found that the vast majority of overeaters can break the "I blew it" syndrome by using these strategies. And almost invariably, my clients who cut off mistakes this way for 24 hours don't gain a pound and typically go on to lose weight that week.

And even more important, they've learned how to stop chain-eating, a major enemy of thin—not just for when they're losing the weight, but for the rest of their lives.

All it takes for most people is to use this technique three or four times! By then you'll find that saying "I blew it" is no longer automatic, but getting back on track is!

The biggest surprise is that this pattern, which has doomed so many to failure for so long, can be broken quickly—with the right strategy. Try it!

KNOW YOUR PATTERN, AND YOU CAN PREDICT YOUR BEHAVIOR

Once you have contained your mistake, it's time to learn from it. As we note many times in this book, there is an amazing amount of predictability in eating behavior. If you know your pattern, you can predict your behavior and develop a plan to control it for the future. And I have learned time and again in my work: *Errors almost always follow a typical pattern.* The same people gain back the same weight with the same foods in the same place at the same time of day (or week) for the same reasons they gave themselves the last time they slipped! It's like Yogi Berra famously said, "It's *déjà vu* all over again."

Look for a pattern. That's number one. I say there is a pattern. You'd be surprised how many clients say there isn't, but after they review the following questions, they smile and say, "Oh, *that!*"

Unlock Your REP (Repeating Eating Pattern)

These questions uncover *your* predictable pattern in eating mistakes. This pattern is important to learn so you can plan the right preventive strategies.

What type of *food?* Was it a sweet or crunchy food? Creamy? A baked good? What food was it exactly that started you off? Do you have a history of abusing a particular food?

What type of *mood?* What kind of state were you in when you made the mistake—nervous, sleep-deprived, bored, stressed, angry, frustrated? Did you tell yourself you were hungry? What reason did you give yourself?

What *environment?* What *place* were you in when you made the mistake? Were you in a restaurant? At the movies, outdoors, a friend's house, your mother's—or was it in your own home? If so, in what room? The kitchen, the dining room, or in front of the TV? Or were you in the office? This is a problematic place for many of us. Unlike at home, you can't control what foods are brought into your place of work. Holiday seasons, grateful clients, conference food, vending machines, the office cafeteria—work tempts you with food you've made a full-time job of keeping out of your home!

What *people* **were you with?** Were you with anyone when your eating went wrong? Friends? Business associates? Family? Also ask: Were you with a large group of people? Studies have shown that *people tend to eat much more with a large group* than when alone or one-on-one. This will alert you to be prepared by eating something before you go out for group meals so you will be less tempted by everyone else's food or by being hungry.

What *time* **was it?** One of the most reliable truths in my work is that eating mistakes have a favored *time of day.* This is what I called the "Cinderella Syndrome" earlier in the book. Knowing when the clock strikes for *you* tells you when it's time to take preventive measures. And also take a look at the *time of the week.* Is *your* Friday Night Fight with heavyweight calories? Do Sunday night blues make you eat more?

10 NO-FAIL STRATEGIES TO PREVENT YOUR EATING MISTAKES

After containing your mistake and finding its pattern, it's time to *work out a strategy to stop it from repeating.* By avoiding the guilt of "I blew it," you've reached this new stage of growth: where you use your slip as a compass to lead you to greater control and success. *Preventing* mistakes is infinitely better than rehabilitation! Successful preventive strategies save you great amounts of energy, frustration, and time.

Strategy #1: Break availability. You can't eat what's not there! All studies show *The more food around; the more food you eat—* and the more you think of food and feel yourself tempted.

- If the "cheat" food is around, get rid of it for the next week(s), even if it hasn't been bothering you.
- If it's for others in your family, *avoid proximity.* Stay away from it. If it's in the office, keep your distance.
- Don't work or have a phone chat in the "Fat Room"(your kitchen).
- Avoid eye contact. Never underestimate the power of the visual! Just seeing some foods makes you want to put them right into your mouth. Put them in a brown bag instead or in foil so

when you open the refrigerator, the sight of them is unavailable to your eyes. Or put them on a high shelf in a cupboard with wooden doors. Take it from its see-through wrapping, and put it in a metal container. In a restaurant, don't "eye" the whole menu, especially not the dessert section.

Strategy #2: Delay. Time is your friend if you're employing strategy. As time passes, cravings pass or other events capture your attention. If you tell yourself you'll eat the fattening food tonight or tomorrow instead of now, most typically when that time comes, you'll have a lot less interest in it. The original desire has usually dissipated.

Strategy #3. Use binge busters. Sometimes you want to end a craving immediately. That's where these easy-to-carry products come in handy.

- **Sugar Blocker Gum.** This gum is the most effective craving killer. It deactivates the sweet receptors on the tongue. After chewing for 10 minutes, anything sweet that you eat will no longer have a sweet taste, but rather, an unpleasant taste. And anything else you eat for the next half hour has very little or a bitter taste. Some of my clients who don't even like sweets use this gum because the unpleasant taste it creates in the mouth kills all cravings and appetite so you have no desire to eat.
- **Halls Sugar-Free Mentho-Lyptus drops.** These mentholated cough drops can be found in almost any drugstore in the world. Just one overwhelms your taste buds and sense of smell. Walk into a room with pizza, and it won't have the same tempting aroma. Even the sight of it won't be appealing. There is no 5-minute wait with these drops, so when you need instant help, reach for these.
- **Listerine Breath Strips (or a comparable brand).** These flavored breath strips melt on your tongue, are very easy to find, and act immediately. They may or may not be stronger for you than the Halls drops. The key is to buy whichever has the sharpest taste for you and kills the desire to eat. Many of my clients put one or two of these on their tongue while they wait for their food in a restaurant, so they don't touch the breadbasket, or they use them to kill a craving anytime they feel tempted or hungry.

Strategy #4: Don't go hungry. Success on a diet is not about being hungry. Getting hungry is usually not related to proper diet but to poor planning. But don't confuse hunger with boredom or listlessness or the "habit hunger" you feel doing something you traditionally associate with eating, such as watching TV. Genuine hunger usually starts when you are approaching 3 to 4 hours without eating a healthy snack or meal. Here are six surefire strategies winners use to not go hungry.

- **Flood your appetite.** Most people don't gain weight from low-calorie *liquid* foods. Nor do they get compulsive about them. For something sweet, have a low-cal sweet *beverage*. A Designer Protein shake or Alba Shake (made with water, diet soda, or coffee) kills appetite and sugar cravings and is nutritious (less than 100 calories). The Jeff's Diet Chocolate or Vanilla soda has a dab of cream and fat-free milk that gives it a rich, creamy texture for only 20 calories per bottle. My heaviest clients have never been able to drink more than two or three without feeling full.

  Carbonated beverages also kill hunger. Carbonation creates a feeling of fullness in the stomach. And typically, carbonated products are cold liquids. The combination of carbonation plus the cold makes a doubly strong appetite suppressor.

  Tomato juice is the ultimate hunger killer because it's a very heavy liquid and typically very flavorful. It's particularly helpful when you're asked at a restaurant if you'd like to order a drink. It's a safe appetite suppressant with very few calories—far less than alcohol or the contents of the breadbasket! For those who like spicy beverages, the "spicy hot" variety of V8 Juice is a sure winner, at fewer than 40 calories.
- **Use temperature control for appetite control.** Extremes of temperature—hot or cold, particularly liquids—make the body feel full immediately and put off feelings of hunger. Try this experiment yourself: Drink two glasses of water, one iced and the other room temperature. You'll find it takes much longer to finish the ice water, and it makes you feel fuller. As many people have discovered, when there's little time to eat, a cup of hot coffee does wonders to take the edge off your

appetite. It'll even save you from picking on the breadbasket when hungry.

Most people would rank *soup* as number one in fixing their appetite. Have a bowl of one of the 70-calorie Tabatchnick frozen vegetable soups. Carry around the instant soups that come in envelopes, such as Lipton Cup-a-Soup (especially the tomato!).

- **Use your binge busters!** Halls Mentho-Lyptus drops, especially, make a powerful appetite killer. But Sugar Blocker Gum and breath strips (such as Listerine) also are reliable hunger stoppers.
- **Eat *the* appetite control cracker.** One cracker has a special place in my armament of antihunger weapons. I have seen more people abuse crackers than be helped by them, particularly the thin, salty, crispy ones. Most have too many carbohydrates and too little fiber. There is one notable exception—the *GG Scandinavian Bran Crispbread.* Only 16 calories and 3 grams of carbohydrates, but a generous 3 grams of fiber. And when you subtract the 3 grams of fiber from the 3 grams of carbohydrates, you get zero net carbs! It's the ultimate "no-carb carb." Two or three of these crackers kill appetite for hours with negligible calories even if you eat several extra throughout the day. All of my clients who use them daily say they are rarely hungry. Even if these crackers aren't available in your health food store, I strongly recommend that you order them (see Resources on page 302). They make great sandwiches with rich fiber, and you can carry them everywhere, so hunger will never again be part of your weight control. And you can search every health food store in America and not find a cracker this thick and crunchy with those low calories and carbs.

My winners carry it everywhere in their briefcases or pocketbooks for a snack or minimeal. Turn it into a pizza with fat-free tomato sauce and fat-free shredded mozzarella; or a dessert with fat-free cream cheese topped with jam or apple butter; or cinnamon toast with no-cal I Can't Believe It's Not Butter spray, cinnamon, and Splenda! (I'll talk about this further in the diet chapter.)

The GG cracker is perfect for people who travel a lot and have irregular hours. Add it to your ThinPack: a self-sealing bag that also contains a low-cal hot chocolate, a Lipton Cup-a-Soup, and Laughing Cow Light Cheese Triangles (which can last a few hours without refrigeration). Carry it with you, or put it in your glove compartment. It's particularly helpful for PMS hunger or when carpooling during meal times.

- **Throw veggies at it!** "Think green and white." Under my program, most green and white vegetables made without fat are free foods. Make yourself half a pound of steamed broccoli with garlic, herbs, and spices. Order steamed Chinese vegetables with scallions and ginger. You can eat all you want.

- **Throw protein at it!** Pick a low-fat, nutritious protein, such as an egg white omelet, grilled shrimp salad, or my egg salad recipe (see page 221).

- **Have a fourth meal or minimeal,** such as two Oscar Meyer or Hebrew National fat-free franks on sauerkraut. Or two pieces of GG Beefsteak Light Rye (40 calories each), a slice of fat-free American cheese (Kraft, Borden's, or Weight Watcher's—30 calories), and a slice of Hillshire Farms ham (just 10 calories). How's that for a toasted ham and cheese sandwich? If you use the GGs, no more calories than a cup of low-fat yogurt or an apple—but a lot more filling!

Strategy #5: Avoid packaging temptation. The colors, wording, and photographs on all food packages have one goal only: to tempt you and increase your hunger for the product. Store packaged foods in brown bags to stop this temptation. Or discard the package entirely, and put the food in an opaque container.

The best way to avoid the temptation of packaging you find especially alluring is to not even go down their aisles in the store, or at least don't stop when you do. And try not to shop in that vulnerable period of late afternoon when the blood sugar dips, or the packaging will look even more tempting. Or should I say *too* tempting?

Strategy #6: Use blocking behaviors. In psychology, the technique called *blocking behavior* is the strategy of doing something *harmless* or positive to make it hard to do some other thing that is *harmful* or negative. This works very well for weight control. For example, at a party, my female winners will carry a clutch purse in one hand and a nonalcoholic drink in the other, stopping their hands from reaching out when fattening hors d'oeuvres come by at a cocktail hour.

Or if junk food is a problem when you turn on TV, block this behavior with a no-eating rule, keep your hands busy with beverages, or chew on gum. Or instead of nuts or chips, dip into a bowl of crunchy vegetables or roasted ones with Cajun spices. Many of my clients take up needlepoint or knitting to keep from eating when they watch TV. If you tend to "pick" while cooking, put veggies on the counter to nibble or sip on an ice-cold beverage with a straw. Or block that behavior entirely by brushing your teeth and leaving a little toothpaste in your mouth. You could even pop a Halls Mentho-Lyptus drop or Listerine Breath Strip. (I suggest you always keep one or both of these items readily available in the

What the Winners Say

When you first begin trying cognitive switching, it might seem artificial, and you have to push yourself to do it. But after a couple of days, it will become as natural for you as it has for my own clients. Think like a winner to cut off and prevent errors.

The food looks so tempting. Do I like it enough to wear it? I've tasted it all before. It didn't make me happy; it only made me fat.

I'll just have one. If I could have just one, why have I been fat for 20 years? I've been eating for decades, and one was never enough. Stop lying to myself. If I don't take the first little taste, if I don't begin, I won't have any problem.

One pretzel won't hurt. I've gained more weight with my fingers than with my mouth. Remember, I'm a chain eater with finger foods.

Those rolls look so good. Stop looking at and glorifying the very food that makes me fat. What am I looking at? I know what rolls look like— I'm wearing 10 pounds of them now. It's not free; I have to wear it.

Those desserts must taste good. Thin tastes better.

I'll feel deprived if I don't have a dessert. The only real deprivation

kitchen or the room you use for preparing food.) You can block the negative behavior or even convert it to a positive by eating healthy instead of fattening!

Strategy #7: Diversion. As talked about previously in this book, *diversion* is a powerful way of getting your mind off your craving by doing an activity you find absorbing or beneficial.

Strategy #8: Cognitive switching. *Cognitive switching* means talking to yourself in a new way.

All of us carry on a continuing internal dialogue about other people or events or about ourselves. How we talk to ourselves about *food* either encourages overeating or empowers us to limit or avoid it entirely. The winners at weight control permanently change their *thinking* as well as their weight. Changing your thinking is necessary to change your behavior. One technique I've developed for this was the subject of my keynote address at the National Weight Control

is never being thin. I've already spent 10 years being fat due to eating desserts. I'm living my life backward. I'm putting a piece of food before my body and my right to be thin and healthy. Was I in paradise when I was eating desserts? No! I was fat and miserable.

I blew it by eating the french fries, so I stopped trying and ate everything. I was very bad! I didn't blow it; I had a break in control. Everyone makes mistakes when learning a new skill. I contain the mistakes and move forward.

Every time I see sweets, I crave them. A craving is a feeling—not a command. Feelings pass. There'll be no pain, no blood loss. I will not have to call 911 for the rescue squad. Studies show that cravings pass in minutes. If I don't negotiate or equivocate, isn't thin worth a few minutes?

I bought it for company, but I ate most of it. Thin starts in the supermarket! If I don't buy it, I don't have to wear it. I'm the easiest client to help; I've gained all my weight in my own kitchen. If I control what I put in that one room, I control my weight.

and Obesity Symposium held at the Columbia-Presbyterian Medical Center a number of years ago. It's called cognitive switching.

You can actually switch your thinking about how you eat by talking to yourself in a new way, then reinforcing it. The cognitive switch of the winners replaces the old, defeatist way of thinking about food that only tempts you to overeat with a new way that matches your goals. (See "What the Winners Say" on page 116 for examples of cognitive switching.)

Strategy #9: Think substitution, not deprivation. The mark of what I call "great substitute" foods is that they are light, delicious alternatives to higher-calorie foods. They have a similar look and texture as their higher-calorie counterparts, and they must taste great too, so they leave you satisfied. They literally give you the taste without the calories. Most of the foods are new to the market and were not even available a few years ago. I'll discuss these foods in greater length in the diet chapter—but right now, here are some examples of how these foods can be helpful.

Every Sunday, Marcy takes her family to a restaurant that's a gathering place for the community. She knows from experience that she has too soft of a spot in her heart for their strawberry shortcake, so she came up with the perfect substitute: fresh strawberries on a Van's Belgian waffle topped with fat-free Reddi-wip! She'd come home and have her own delicious strawberry shortcake for a grand total of fewer than 150 calories and virtually no grams of sugar. She didn't feel deprived one bit!

For a chocolate dessert, have the Skinny Cow Mousse Pop, which looks like a Dove Bar and is as rich as any restaurant dessert.

Flood a craving for something sweet with liquids such as diet hot chocolate (good for PMS). One of my favorite choices is Jeff's Diet Egg Cream (in supermarkets and specialty stores or online at www.getcreamed.com) or the flavored Alba shakes.

Drown a salty craving with Lipton's Instant Tomato Soup or (my favorite) Hot and Spicy V8.

For salty/crunchy cravings—pickles are excellent!

And on page 285, I list the top 25 low-calorie treats that can meet and retreat almost any craving. A lot of these great new foods didn't even exist a few months ago. And most of my clients say that they've made all the difference in wiping out cravings and feelings of deprivation.

Strategy #10: Mental rehearsal. The *mental rehearsal* technique is a powerful preventive strategy when going into a situation with food you know is a major stumbling block for you. I developed this technique exclusively for my clients, and with it, you can actually desensitize yourself *in advance* to the power of that food to tempt you.

My studies in the psychology of learning taught me that the human psyche gets bored quickly with constant repetition. *Mental rehearsal* uses this trick to turn us off to the very foods that tempt us the most.

First, identify what foods you will find the most tempting in terms of sight and smell in the situation you are preparing for. Then repeat to yourself something like this: *I will smell pizza when I walk through the door, or I will smell cookies baking. Or I will see the desserts.* And then tell yourself: *It doesn't work for me. And I don't want to wear it! This is the food that made me fat.* Then put a negative association with the food—your highest weight, a part of your body where you can't stand the fat. Imagine the food going to your thighs, your derriere, or a bloated face the next day. Imagine the bulging stomach such foods have given you.

Keep repeating it till you get bored with the repetition and you say to yourself, *Enough already!* The whole thing takes just 1 to 3 minutes. Most of my clients can do it in a minute. What it does is reprogram your mind against the two strongest elements of cravings: seeing and smelling. So when you walk into the situation, the food won't have that magnetic pull on you any longer. All of us who have gone into a beautiful restaurant, affair, or party know what it's like to look at something and think, *Wow, that looks interesting.* Mental rehearsal takes away that "wow effect." The few minutes it takes can save you thousands of calories and endless days and hours in the gym!

We all have power over the feeling of deprivation—
the ability to control it, decrease it, even extinguish it—
because the source of it begins and ends within you.

The Eighth Thin Commandment:
Stop Feeling Deprived

COMMANDMENT ESSENTIALS

- Change your mindset—not just your eating habits.
- Learn to Thinspeak (supporting yourself with motivational, not demoralizing, words).
- Reward yourself with a new outfit or piece of jewelry instead of food.
- Let your old trigger foods go, and embrace the delicious foods that won't put you at war with yourself.
- Remember, thin tastes better.
- Record and then regularly listen to an empowerment tape to help you think and feel like a weight-control winner.

DO YOU RECOGNIZE YOURSELF in this scenario? You've been dieting for several weeks. Your clothes are getting looser. You're seeing more definition in your face. You have more stamina. You're getting compliments about how great you look and how much weight you've lost. And then, you start getting sloppy. You begin snacking again at night, dipping into the nuts or chips or chocolate candies, or you return to skipping meals or picking at the breadbasket. You've worked so hard, you're approaching your goal, you're almost there . . . and then you sabotage yourself, and the pounds start rolling back, or your weight loss comes to a crashing halt as you create a plateau with the extra calories. For others, the backslide may come a little later, when they are on maintenance.

This point in the weight-control process—the threshold of achievement—is one of the most critical spots you'll encounter when losing weight or trying to keep it off, a place where you're most likely to relapse into old eating habits. Call it "diet burnout" or whatever you want, but at this point, with success at hand, many people find themselves saying, "I don't feel like doing this anymore. I'm missing out on the fun. It's not fair. Everybody else is eating it."

Sound familiar? Take a look at your own food history. How many times before have you returned to the foods, places, or behaviors that torpedoed your efforts at weight loss right out of the water? And how often was it because you felt that you were being deprived of your favorite goodies and treats, and you felt you wanted to eat "normally"?

Frequently, with my clients, I point out that this is the only area of their lives where they've never learned to live with success. Just as they begin to taste victory, they return to old behaviors. "What's wrong with me? Why do I keep doing this again and again?" they often ask.

IS THIN WORTH 5 MILLION DOLLARS?

Rose, a financial executive, came to see me after many years of successfully losing weight and then, invariably, regaining it. She was just turning 40, and she didn't want to start another decade of her life repeating the same pattern of yo-yo dieting. For the past 20 years, every morning she'd awoken thinking about her weight, dreading the moment when she had to face her closet and decide what she would wear for the day. Rose didn't even keep any full-length mirrors in her home. She found it depressing to see her own reflection.

"I'm not as rich as some of the people I work with on Wall Street," she told me at our first session, "but through the deals I've brokered, I've managed to save about 5 million dollars—and I'd gladly give it all away to end this struggle in my life. I feel confident that I know how to make more money, but I don't know how I can lose my weight and keep it off."

Part of the reason that accomplished and successful women like Rose and so many others falter and return to self-defeating eating patterns is because, although they've lost the weight many times, they've never changed their thinking. Dieting is a pain-motivated goal. We go on diets because we're unhappy, but as soon as we drop a few pounds, we become happier and motivation fades. But that's only half the story. We might all rally a little more motivation and commitment, and we might stick with our diets till the end if only—if only we didn't feel we were missing something.

This sense of deprivation is the mindset behind the behaviors—it's the self-talk that generates the actions. It often flies under the radar, eluding our awareness completely, but it's the greater problem. This is the underlying thinking that says any guidelines are *bad*—you should be able to eat it all and *still* be thin. This way of thinking is akin to a child who has to have everything he sees and doesn't care about the consequences.

Dieting has always been associated with deprivation. The two words resonate together like flip sides of the same coin. Yet in 2005, that's old thinking. A central goal of this book is to prove to you, through the foods and "five-star recipes" that I've given in the food chapter, that dieting is no longer about deprivation, but about sub-stitution. My many clients, an exceptionally blessed group of people who frequently travel the world, attend glamorous dinner parties, and dine in the great mansions and finest restaurants around the globe, have chosen all of their favorite low-calorie foods, and I'm happy to pass along a list of their choices to you. They've tasted it all, and I'll dare to say their endorsement is as trustworthy as that of the toughest food reviewer. The selections they've named are the best of the best substitutes available today, and many of them are included in my ABC Eating Plan (see page 175), which will show you how to enjoy gourmet meals while still losing weight. Today, with so many restau-rants serving light entrées and low-calorie selections, dining out is never a problem either. My clients don't complain that they can't lead lives of normal eating. On the contrary, they're surprised at how easy it is to make the transition to a diet that includes delicious foods and gives creative strategies for dining at the best restaurants and parties.

Although changes in food culture have been taking place, and all of these great products have been coming into the marketplace over the past 3 or 4 years, the programming and the mindset about deprivation has been in place in the human psyche for many years, even decades, and it won't be easily displaced without a conscious effort. Other diet programs don't deal with it. They don't discuss managing feelings of deprivation or suggest strategies to prevent them. However, my clients and I have spent a large percentage of our time together examining this phenomenon over the years. Our conclusion? *Overcoming the deprivation mindset is a key and critical dynamic for success at weight control.*

Deprivation is triggered by behaviors, thinking, and, on occasion, failing to act. Sometimes, we even think and behave in ways that fuel it. Mastering deprivation means changing both your thinking and your behavior. It also means learning the techniques and skills that will help you defuse and even defeat the deprivation mindset. In this chapter, I'll take you through the steps and show you how to . . .

1. Change the mindset that's generating the behaviors

2. Use strategies to minimize or prevent feelings of deprivation

3. Deal with deprivation issues head-on

4. Go beyond deprivation to liberation

THE DEEDS THAT DEFEAT YOU

Before you bought this book and started learning about this program, you had all of the foods you wanted, whenever you wanted them, but that freedom didn't make you happy—it only made you heavy! If you're like most people, the truth is, the more you eat, the worse you feel. And chances are that you bought this book to be rescued from the foods that have made you heavy again and again. Nevertheless, you most likely still fear the idea of being separated from the pleasure of dining—the whole concept of dieting is still imprinted on your psyche as deprivation.

Why is it so easy to feel deprived? Because people want immediacy—now! Although the goals for weight loss are long-term, they are actually pretty short-lived on the scale of life's problems. Most people on a diet can start to see noticeable changes in 10 to 30 days. After 90 days, the results will show dramatically. You don't have to get to the final goal to start seeing a payoff. The moment you experience the first signs of improvement, you're at a turning point in the process of weight loss—and this stage is easily undermined and overwhelmed by the deprivation mindset. To start wavering is human.

When temptations and cravings come into the picture, it's a high-risk, full-alert food situation for anyone who is trying to watch her weight. Giving in, giving yourself the "gift" of this "treat" feels normal. Denying it to yourself makes you feel deprived. Some individuals even suffer from what I call the "Eve Complex," the tendency to feel an even greater desire for something that is restricted or forbidden, just as Eve had everything but couldn't resist the forbidden fruit in the Garden of Eden.

Don't blame yourself for responding this way. It's basic: When something gives us pleasure, we want to return to it again and again. In this way, we're no different from any creature in the animal kingdom. This is the pleasure principle that pushes human behavior on the most fundamental level. But we do have one advantage—an intervening variable—the ability to be aware of the cost and consequences of our choices.

Of course, your favorite foods taste good, and they're delicious; that's why you love them—until a few minutes after they're down the hatch.

By definition, it's almost impossible for most middle-class people to be truly *deprived* of food. Indeed, the opposite is true; we're drowning in an overabundance of food. Recent World Health Organization statistics indicated that for the first time in human history, the number of people who are overweight exceeds the number of people who are underfed or starving. Children living in poverty are deprived. Families trapped in war-torn cities are deprived. Prisoners on starvation rations are deprived. But the fact is, if you have an interest or need to read this book, I'm fairly sure you can eat anything you want, anytime you want. The ultimate decision to eat or not to eat is always yours.

Objectively, the state of deprivation may be a myth, but the feeling is very real. What many people don't realize is that it's also a learned response. And what has been learned can be unlearned. *We all have power over the feeling of deprivation. You have the ability to control it, decrease it, even extinguish it, because the source of it begins and ends within you.*

By becoming aware and zeroing in on your own thinking and behavior, you can eliminate the causes and the processes that ignite deprivation. You may not realize it, but your thoughts trigger your deprivation, which in turn triggers your behavior. Change your thoughts, learn a new response, practice it until it becomes automatic, and you will, at last, stop fueling your own deprivation. You'll cut it off, nip it in the bud, release yourself from the prison of being controlled by food, and be free to get on with the business of getting—and living—trim. The winners who have come to this realization no longer feel deprived, but liberated.

THE THOUGHTS THAT MISLEAD YOU

The diet advice that abounds on bookstore shelves and in magazines doesn't discuss the deprivation mindset because most professionals in the field aren't trained to address changing thinking and feeling. But with my background in psychology and my study of the motivational techniques of the advertising world, I've been heavily influenced about how to change thinking—and how to replace nonproductive behaviors with behaviors that are productive.

This is the essence of good therapy of all kinds, including weight therapy, and any weight program that doesn't deal with an individual's underlying mental and emotional orientations will be inadequate. Since most diet plans are exclusively about the right foods, right calories, and right carbohydrates, it's clear why we have such a high rate of failure. Most programs are doomed because they omit the principal motivators and determinants of successful human behavior. As I have said before, diets are just words on a page—acting and succeeding on them is all about the right behavior and the right motivation.

Changing the feelings of deprivation is beyond the scope of the current thinking in the field, but for me and my clients, it's at the core of our efforts. We work intensely together to make the critical shift in thinking.

It's not enough just to change your habits, your mindset has to change too.

Throughout this book, one of my core messages is about the need to abandon childhood food thinking. Here, again, it's important to understand that adult behavior is about making choices. As we grow older, we have a restricted calorie budget. We have to make smart food choices, and over time, it becomes harder to distinguish our food choices from our life choices. Breaking with the psychology of dieting and its association with deprivation is a profound growth step.

Only children think they can have it all. And if they don't, they

(continued on page 128)

9 Behaviors That Increase a Feeling of Deprivation

In a survey of my clients, here are the actions that they find the most important to avoid—and, when counteracted, some of the best ways to ensure success.

1. **Allowing too much proximity.** Keeping all the foods that tempt you around and on display at home fuels a sense of deprivation. Even if you don't eat it, being near a favorite food, just knowing it's in the next room, creates a mental tug-of-war. It's always on your mind, particularly if it's clearly visible. In public settings, "no proximity" means try not to sit near or make eye contact with foods that tempt you. *Control your food curiosity.* Don't go grazing in "food temples" such as supermarkets or gourmet food stores, don't read the sections of a menu with foods you are trying to avoid, and don't survey the dessert tables, hors d'oeuvres, or other foods that tempt you. Remember that the more you center your life on a vulnerability, the more vulnerable your life will become! Availability stimulates craving—it's that simple!

2. **Telling yourself that if you can't have it, you'll be deprived.** Behind this statement is the assumption that *it's not normal; everyone else is having it.* But over the years, everyone who's said this to me has overlooked one obvious truth: Their weight has never been normal because of the foods they're so worried about missing out on. I tell them to worry more about a normal weight, a normal life, normal health, and normal sizes than what everyone else is eating.

3. **Going too long without eating.** If you're starving, just seeing and smelling food will have a powerful impact.

4. **Going into food situations unprepared.** A simple truth of behavior is that if people don't have the right foods around them, eventually they'll eat the wrong ones. If you go into a conference room meeting for a day, and muffins and cookies or other foods that are a problem for you are being served, and you haven't brought your ThinPack of low-calorie snacks along, you will eat what is there, or you will feel a constant struggle with temptation.

5. **Forgetting that you know what it tastes like.** You've already tasted it all; there are no more surprises. You know the taste and texture of virtually every food imaginable—what more can it give you?

6. **Tasting trigger foods that you've**

decided to Box Out. Don't forget that you can't have "just a little" of the foods that have been a problem for you historically. As I've discussed many times in this book, taking a taste of a trigger food may reactivate your cravings and unleash your thinking, looking, and obsessing about it. Invariably, tasting foods that you have decided to Box Out makes it harder, because the pleasure principle of the human psyche makes you want to finish it and have more and not be a "taster." It's not about the calories in a taste but about the cravings and food interest that taste reactivates.

7. **Not giving yourself alternative rewards.** You can minimize your deprivation response before entering a risky food situation by doing a Mental Rehearsal and reminding yourself of your new reward system—both are very effective uses of psychology. Tell yourself that you won't eat the french fries, but you'll buy yourself a beautiful outfit, you'll do something you love, or you'll be able to wear a favorite outfit that doesn't fit right now. This technique is a favorite among my clients.

8. **Failing to embrace the substitutes.** In today's food culture, the choices for low-calorie, low-fat foods are so vast, there are enough to accommodate every personal taste and preference. Studies show that if you don't have your favorite food, but you have your second favorite, you're better able to control it. For example, my clients who love chocolate cookies find that chocolate mousse is very satisfying, but without the crunch that would trigger compulsive overeating.

9. **Forgetting that eating a food is not free.** Once you realize the high cost of a behavior, it reduces the attractiveness of that behavior—meaning that eating a food that sabotages your weight loss or your control is not a "treat" but a costly decision. Don't confuse a "great taste" with a "great life." The major reason you have been miserable or unhappy with your weight is because of these types of foods. See yourself at your highest weight, and ask yourself the powerful question that breaks any feeling of deprivation: "Do I like it enough to wear it?" When you realize the fact that you may already be wearing several pounds of this food, ask yourself, "Do I really need another serving of such a 'treat'?"

are therefore deprived. Yet this is the same thinking that envelops the weight-loss industry. This is what we are being led to believe. As I've explained before, some leading diet experts are the chief reinforcers of the myth that if you're denied something, you'll binge. By now it should be no big surprise to see me write again that when it comes to trigger foods, once you stop eating them and keeping them around, you lose a great deal if not all of your cravings. And most people don't miss them once they realize the true cost of eating them. Although it may be difficult at first to let go of trigger foods, the long-

Sample Tape #2: Keeping the Winners' Edge

To begin your tape, name the specific foods that have caused you to feel deprived. Think about what has happened to your weight when these foods are in your life. Then proceed with the rest of the dialogue.

- "Today, I will stay focused on what is essential, and I will not waste my time on what is nonessential. I will have flipped the switch that turns off the thoughts of deprivation in my head. I've seen it all and tasted it all in the world of food. I can succeed at being trim. Each time I say, 'No, thank you,' I say, 'yes,' to being trim and successful. Only the thin say, 'No, thank you.' To be in control is empowering. To have the power to say, 'No, thank you,' to that which has destroyed my figure (or control) again and again is liber-

ating. I don't need to look at it, think about it, or taste it. I've had enough for three lifetimes."

- Emphasize why you had your weight problem. "Yes, this food (name it) has a pleasant taste for a few moments, but these few moments have cost me years, decades of misery. It's just a piece of food. Don't be a "food whiner" and make yourself miserable. You can have all you want, whenever you want, but you'll never have the life you want.

- "By taking it one day at a time, I'm building a lifetime of being in control. If I find myself obsessing about a piece of food, I will tell myself, "Get over it; you're already wearing it. If it made you so happy, why were you always so miserable about your weight?"

- "I will remember all that I want to

term benefits far outweigh any short-term discomforts. My clients
and I have found that it is easier to say "no" than to just have a little.

A Tale of Two Closets

My client, Martha, a charismatic young travel agent from Chicago,
had lost weight and regained it so often that she had several sets of
clothing, one in her favorite size, the others in increasingly larger
sizes. Fortunately, she had two closets in her bedroom. She kept her
preferred clothes in one and her wardrobe of larger sizes in the other.

do, and I won't worry about any
foods that may divert me. I don't
live in a fairyland where I can have
it all and still be trim, but that
doesn't mean I'm deprived. I have
so much going for me; I deserve to
be in control. I deserve to be trim. I
deserve to succeed in the world of
food. I won't let my PMS, or the
Poor Me Syndrome, block my
memory and make me forget that
when I had it all, I ate it all, and I
was miserable. Being in control
with my weight and my food makes
me feel empowered each day, makes
me feel better about myself, and
makes me look better. Complacency is the enemy of thin. Letting
myself get sloppy because of the
compliments I'm getting is to not
understand that every time people
say to me how great I look, how

much weight I lost, they're also
thinking how fat I was before. If I
let the compliments go to my head,
they'll soon grow silent again as I
regain the weight."

- "Every so often, I may just see or
smell a food that tempts me. I'll say to
myself, 'It's just for the moment,' because I'm just seeing/smelling it. It's
just a feeling, not a command. Feelings pass, but the taste of thin/trim
can endure for a lifetime when I say,
'No thanks,' to this food(s). It doesn't
work for me, that's why . . . I don't
begin; I don't have any problem!"

- "In eating this way, I will look years
younger. I will feel more attractive
and more empowered as a person.
There are curveballs in life, and although being thin doesn't guarantee
I'll be happy, it does guarantee that I
won't be unhappy because I'm fat."

One morning, she opened the wrong closet by mistake. That day, she needed to dress in one of her larger outfits, since her weight had been creeping up for several weeks. But when she opened the wrong closet and caught a glimpse of all the pretty, stylish clothes that she would much rather be wearing and could not, she slammed the door immediately—hard.

"It was at that moment," she told me later, "I realized that the true deprivation came *from* eating all of the foods that had caused my weight to balloon. My behavior had *deprived me* of wearing the clothes I loved."

The insight that had hit Martha, which she helped me to see when she shared her story, is that we experience liberation only when we are free to live as we choose, not as hostages to a piece of food, taking orders from cravings and suffering from a gnawing feeling that we're missing out on something.

Today, both of Martha's closets hold clothing in the same ideal size. When she thinks back to her former "fat closet," she thinks: "Never again." She enjoys wearing her beautiful clothes and looking her best, and she knows she'll always have the strategies to keep her in control—and liberated!

BACK TALK THAT WORKS

Deprivation doesn't just happen; it's something that is done to you. The feelings that you've experienced on previous diets, of missing out on something, were produced by the programming of your past, the prerecorded mindset, which you, in turn, perpetuate and impose on yourself. Whenever you are near food, the old tape switches on, and these messages go to work fostering your feelings of deprivation and eroding your control over food.

Most of my clients find it easy to see the effects of this programming when they are in my office. They realize that foods that consistently trigger overeating or endless cravings are enemies, not treats. They know that the real deprivation is in never living trim. But self-talk isn't always conscious or even rational. It was "taped" long ago and reinforced ever since. As a result, even the most logical and determined dieters can find themselves thinking, "I can't live without it," when they know perfectly well there is nothing essential to survival in a candy bar or a potato chip.

It will make me feel better. It will make me happy. It will comfort me. This thinking is at the core of the deprivation mindset, and the greatest thing you can do is to eclipse these thoughts and connect to a new voice. A food that you enjoy for comfort shouldn't bring you discomfort.

Learning to rewrite your internal dialogue can be the difference between success and failure. It can speed you along the road away from the deprivation mindset, or it can drag you back and keep you enslaved to your trigger foods. The choice is yours, because with time and practice, you can erase your old self-talk and replace it with positive, realistic messages. Those who succeed at weight control engage in a supportive inner dialogue. Simply put, their words to themselves are motivating, not demoralizing, and when they're faced with old programming, they dare to talk back. So can you. Here are a few sample retorts to get you started.

LEARNING TO THINSPEAK

I'm missing out on the fun.	What fun? You had it for years, and it didn't make you happy; it only made you fat.
Everybody's eating it.	True or not, you've had enough for three lifetimes.
What's wrong with a taste?	Taking a taste makes it harder. (Most people can taste most foods, but as I've discussed at length, some individuals have a long history of abusing a single food or type of food. In these cases, it's easier to rule out the food entirely. Taking a taste is like an ex-smoker taking a cigarette. It's restarting the pattern. It's better not to think about it at all, much like getting over a failed love affair. Take a taste only if your history indicates you have been a "taster" with this food; otherwise, avoid it.)
I just want it.	I want to be thin even more. I don't want it enough to wear it.
It's so hard.	Being fat is harder.

If you don't do the strategies, if you go too long without eating, and if you don't eat low-calorie substitutes, it *will* seem hard. If you think you can't or that you have to give up the pleasure of fine food for a lifetime, it will seem *impossibly* hard. But hopefully, all the lessons in this book have already convinced you that being thin isn't about giving up the fun in your life or the pleasure of great dining—it's about giving up sloppy compulsive eating behaviors and habits that keep you from succeeding.

Turning Off the Deprivation Switch

Deprivation is a learned experience—most of the people on earth have never seen or tasted the majority of the foods that many of us "can't live without." It's a learned cultural experience. *And what can be learned can be unlearned* is a central theme of this book.

One of the most efficient ways to deprogram yourself is to make a tape. When you're feeling deprived, the mechanism busily at work within you is the voice in your head. In a way, you're subjecting yourself to self-hypnosis: "I have to have it. I have to have it. If I don't, I'm deprived."

It's one thing to understand this intellectually, but it's dramatically more effective to enhance what you know through the power of listening to a tape or CD, which will instill a new message into your subconscious—and you actually feel it!

Use this tool to turn off the feelings of deprivation. Counteract them. Give yourself a new internal dialogue.

There are two major reasons that my clients don't find the work we do together hard. One is strategy. The other is that they don't feel deprived. You can have the same benefits by making a tape for yourself. It's not required, but it will make it easier to defeat the deprivation mindset. If you choose not to tape, you can get some of the same effects by writing key statements from the sample script on Post-its and putting them up around your home. Being a winner is a matter of thinking and feeling like a winner. You can get all the lessons simply from reading this book, but you can get them more quickly and effectively if you make yourself a tape. Realize that you're listening to a tape already, every day, running through your head. This strategy just substitutes a new tape full of empowering visions for you and your life so that you can think like a winner.

You can eat like a millionaire in the world of calories and still look like a million.

The Ninth Thin Commandment:
Treat Your Calories Like Dollars

COMMANDMENT ESSENTIALS

- Eat high-calcium dairy foods and cinnamon, both of which make fat cells behave more efficiently.
- Substitute delicious light versions of your favorite foods for calorie-laden "fat" versions.
- Drink 16 ounces of water to help keep calories and carbs from being stored as fat.
- Watch for hidden calories, such as the right foods being prepared the wrong way.
- Spend your calories only on foods you really care about.
- Eat foods that provide high satiety, but low calories.

YOU'RE IN THE STORE BUYING ALUMINUM FOIL. Two brands of similar quality have the same price, but one reads: "30 percent more free!" Which one would you choose?

So would I.

We deeply respect our money and with good reason. We work hard and only have so much. No one needs to be told: "Get the biggest bang for your buck."

We also need to respect our *calories*. Your body works hard to burn them, and when you overspend, you have to wear them. Indeed, for most of us, calories cost more than money: in larger-size clothes, medical bills, discomfort, depression, and life expectancy. The good news is that you already have the know-how to profit from your calories: You can *approach weight control simply as an accounting issue, like balancing your checkbook. Treat your calories like dollars, and get the biggest banquet for your buck!*

CALORIENOMICS: STRETCHING YOUR CALORIE DOLLAR

Calorienomics is the strategy of treating your calories like dollars. *You want to get greater value for less cost.* The goal of calorienomics is to be able to eat more food while lessening the calories but not the pleasure of eating—and still lose weight! How's that for a diet plan you can live with?

One of the comments I hear from my clients again and again is that they're eating much more than they were before—and more frequently! And they wonder, especially at the start, if they'll ever lose weight this way.

You wouldn't be reading this book if they didn't.

The secret is that they're also eating more *wisely*—according to the principles of calorienomics. And many also say they're eating with as much or *greater* enjoyment than they did with the foods that made them gain weight.

Just as salary or income determines a budget, certain factors contribute to your body's calorie budget. While genetics sets the lower limit for our weight, *we* set the upper limit by how we spend our calories. Genetics, food choices, and how much you move—these factors give your body *a fixed budget*. It varies from person to person, but *each of us has a given number of calories to spend*. And if you're reading this book, you're having trouble living within your calorie budget, and you want to know the best way to readjust your spending. But—just as with your economic budget—you don't want to sacrifice needlessly or do without the things you care about most.

All of us would like to have it all—but it isn't possible. It would be great to walk into any store and buy whatever we want, but that's not a realistic scenario. Who can walk into Barney's or Wal-Mart and spend a whole paycheck on an outfit when the rent or a mortgage is due?

But often the people who buy so thoughtfully will nibble mindlessly on whatever's in front of them or blow almost a week's weight loss on a bowl of cashews. The same meticulous people who pore over bank statements for unnecessary costs don't think to wonder what outrageous calories lie hidden in a salad dressing or restaurant sauce. The same ones who clip coupons or comparison-shop don't realize what calorie bargains there are in the world of delicious foods. These behaviors give new meaning to that old English saying: "Penny-wise, pound-foolish"!

We don't want to be like the child in the toy store having a tantrum because he can't have all he sees, feeling deprived and missing out on all the goodies. Calorienomics uses your adult budget skills and common sense to stretch your calorie dollar in ways that allow you to have the *foods* as well as the size and figure you love.

Four principles guide calorienomics:

1. Finding foods that are low in calories but high in taste, nutrition, and satiety (how full they make you feel).

2. Finding foods the body uses in a way that promotes greater loss of weight than other foods with equal calories. These "body-friendly" foods either kill appetite with small amounts or give you few calories with large amounts.

3. Finding the very best light substitutes for your favorite foods with the taste, texture, look, and satisfaction of the originals. They keep the taste without the calories.

4. Avoiding the foods and *behaviors* that bust your budget and participating in behaviors that *stretch* it.

The goal of calorienomics is to give you the freedom to *eat more and lose more.* Many diets like to promise that, but calorienomics shows you how to *do* it—easily and simply. Like a good budget that enables a well-rounded life, calorienomics respects the biological *and* social role of food in our lives as well as the need of the psyche for volume, rich taste, and texture. The diet plan you'll find in our food chapter (see page 175) was designed to meet these very goals:

delicious meals and snacks that give you great taste and volume with less calories, that make the body burn calories more efficiently, and that end hunger and cravings. Our calorienomic food plan also helps you painlessly save up calories for those special foods you love as well as the special celebrations you enjoy over food.

Like all of the other commandments in this book, calorienomics provides you with a complete strategy for enjoying your life at a weight that makes you look good and feel good.

THE BUDGET STRETCHERS

You've probably heard it said, "A calorie is a calorie." That may be true in laboratory research, where a calorie is a unit for measuring heat. But in looking at how calories affect weight loss and appetite, some calories are clearly "more equal than others." *Some calories work more efficiently than others in lowering weight or controlling appetite.*

It takes calories to burn calories, and some require more burning than others to get digested and absorbed. And some calories quench appetite, whereas others stimulate it. There are also calories that control appetite and cravings by keeping insulin levels stable. By choosing your calories wisely, you can optimize the body's processes for weight loss without losing taste or volume. These budget stretchers biologically frustrate fat while meeting your psychological needs for satiety and the pleasure of foods you enjoy.

Budget Stretcher #1: The Thermogenic Effect of Food. Food gives calories, but also takes them away. Digestion requires energy, and calories are what the body burns for energy. The amount of caloric energy it takes to break down any given food is called its *thermogenic effect.* This effect accounts for 5 to 10 percent of your metabolic rate, which can make a critical difference in boosting weight loss and maintaining it.

Lean protein has the most thermogenic effect of all foods. It is estimated to use up roughly 30 percent of its calories for digestion. Simple carbohydrates such as baked goods, bagels, or regular white pasta have poor thermogenic effects, burning around 6 to 8 percent of their calories in thermogenesis. Fat calories are the lowest, burning about 3 percent of their calories before going straight to storage (usually on your hips!).

The four thermogenic winners that really exercise your metabolism and work hardest to end your appetite are: White-meat fish and seafood; vegetables that are high-fiber and low-starch; egg whites; and fiber.

But you can eat more of the thermogenic foods that are lower in calories per ounce than the high-carb grains. An egg white omelet, for example, with spinach and mushrooms gives you a complete meal for about the calories of half a cup of brown rice. And I have clients who snack on a pound of green beans (20 calories/ounce) every day, and they still lose weight. But I don't think they'd have the same success with a pound of whole grain pasta or brown rice (more than 100 calories/ounce). While whole grains are certainly nutritious, people often have problems with their quantities. This poses a behavioral problem for weight-control success, particularly when a cup of pasta, rice, or other grains amounts to about the size of a tennis ball, and most people will eat much more than that amount in the real world.

The perfect solution to getting the benefit of grain without the danger of volume is the unique GG Scandinavian Bran Crispbread I describe earlier in this book and in the food chapter (see page 175). For a fraction of the calories, it gives you as much fiber as the best grains plus large volume. Great crunch . . . and for you carb watchers, zero net carbs per serving—find a pasta, rice, or even another cracker that can do that!

Budget Stretcher #2: Foods That Make Fat Cells Behave More Efficiently. Imagine the bonus of a food that comes in wide variety, has great taste, promotes weight loss, kills appetite, and burns fat instead of storing it! In studies that give the same amount of calories to two groups of dieters, the group that gets this food *loses 70 percent more weight* than the group that doesn't. The research shows that this product particularly is good for a trim waistline and a flat stomach. Plus, it's available in every supermarket! What's this "70 percent-edge food?" High-calcium dairy foods.

And there's also a food with *zero* calories that helps weight loss, kills your appetite, and stabilizes your blood sugar with less than a teaspoon of it per day. This food is a delicious spice—cinnamon.

We discuss both these foods at length—as well as how to use them creatively to promote weight loss *and* great dining—in the food chapter.

Budget Stretcher #3: Substitution. Let's face it, in the real world, many of the foods we love are high in calories.

Indeed, many of the foods that are *worst* for us and our weight control have a great taste. We want to lose weight, but not the pleasure of that taste.

Food manufacturers have received much blame for America's obesity problem, but now they are becoming part of the *solution*. Their intense research into what foods people crave the most are resulting in delicious light versions. They are cutting calories, carbs, and fat dramatically out of everything from dressings and snack foods to chocolate truffles and outrageously delicious chocolate mousses. These days, even fast-food chains are coming to our rescue. Wherever you are in the country—in the *world*—you can probably find a fast-food chain outlet that has found a tasty, light-calorie substitute for high-cal fattening meals.

Budget Stretcher #4: Satiety. Certain foods fill you up quickly, so you don't have to eat very much, yet you're not hungry. In a recent satiety study, of all the foods tested, which two stood alone at the top of the list? Fish was right up there with the boiled potato! Beating out the grains, the breads—even oatmeal.

Budget Stretcher #5: Can a Fruit Help You Lose an Extra 10 Pounds? For years, supporters of grapefruit diets have contended that eating that citrus fruit was a surefire way to lose weight.

Now, new research has confirmed their claim. A study at one of the nation's leading hospitals, the Scripps Clinic's Nutrition and Metabolic Research Center, has revealed that people eating three servings of grapefruit a day with their meals lost 3 to 5 pounds a month *without changing their existing diet*. Many patients lost more than 10 pounds.

The study participants consumed three servings of grapefruit a day, in the form of either 8 ounces of grapefruit juice, half a grapefruit, or special capsules of freeze-dried grapefruit with meals. The group that ate the fresh grapefruit lost an average of 3.6 pounds in 30 days, the juice drinkers lost 3.3 pounds, and the participants who took the capsules lost 2.4 pounds.

The researchers conjecture that the chemical properties of grapefruit reduce insulin levels and promote weight loss. The importance of this link may have to do with the hormone's function in weight management. While weight management is not its primary function, insulin assists with the regulation of fat metabolism. So the smaller the insulin spike after a meal, the more efficiently the body processes food for use as energy and the less calories are stored as fat in the body. Grapefruit may possess unique chemical properties that reduce the insulin levels that encourage weight loss.

Ken Fujioka, M.D., principal researcher at the Nutrition and Metabolic Research Center, said, "Whether it's the properties of grapefruit or its ability to satiate appetites, grapefruit appeared to help with weight loss and decreased insulin levels, leading to better health."

What is most significant about the study is that the patients lost the weight without otherwise changing their diet. This debunks the longstanding axiom that a calorie is just a calorie, and all calories are the same. Obviously, the calories of some foods work better than others for weight loss purposes, and this study suggests that grapefruit should be added to the list of calorie stretchers.

The study was reported in January 2004, and it came to my attention as I was preparing this chapter. While I am just beginning to test this "budget stretcher" in my own practice, I wanted to share this late-breaking new research with you.

(*Note:* Individuals taking heart medication should not consume grapefruit with their medication. Please check with your physician on how many hours should elapse between taking your heart medication and eating grapefruit.)

Budget Stretcher #6: Water—The Magic Elixir. The effects of water on weight may not be fully understood or appreciated as of 2005, but it has always been my observation that *water promotes weight loss.*

Most dieters don't drink enough water. To metabolize 1 gram of carbohydrate, for example, your body needs 3 grams of fluid. So drinking enough water can help keep your carbs from being stored as fat. One study suggests that water suppresses appetite, but it's better to drink before a meal than wash your food through your body with large amounts during the meal. Another very recent study shows that after two glasses of water, your system "shifts into high gear and starts burning fat." And German researchers found that people who consume two 8-ounce glasses of water increased their rate of calorie burning by 30 percent about 40 minutes later, and it stayed elevated for more than an hour. Think strategy and drink the water 40 to 60 minutes before a meal so you'll have the calories of the meal more efficiently metabolized. The researchers estimate that drinking eight 8-ounce glasses of water a day—the minimum recommended amount—could burn off an extra 35,000 calories a year, or 10 pounds. There is also evidence that reasonable amounts of *cold* water make your metabolism burn calories to warm you back up (because cold water lowers your body temperature). Elington Darden, Ph.D., author of *Living Longer Stronger,* says "Drinking more ice cold water causes more heat transfer throughout the skin," which indicates calorie-burning. (He goes on to say that even "staying cool instead of being hot will facilitate fat loss two and three times over and above the normal rate.")

Proper hydration helps you with your weight program in other ways. When you begin a diet, your body loses fluid as well as weight. Without adequate fluid, you're more prone to water retention and constipation, which can keep your scale from accurately reflecting your weight loss. In addition, dehydration can make you feel weak or headachy, which in turn can make you want to move and exercise less as well as eat more for additional energy. When dehydrated, all your body systems slow down, so it's good to monitor your body's hydration. Use what I call "the color test": Make sure your urine is white to straw-colored by midday. Then you'll know your body has adequate fluid to conduct its normal calorie-burning processes.

The exact role of water in promoting weight loss is not entirely clear—all the information is not yet in. Some weight specialists believe it may not be a significant factor; others believe it is. All I can share with you is that over the years, I've heard thousands of clients saying, "When I drink more water, I lose more weight." Just don't be excessive; six to eight glasses seems to be adequate for healthy people. Just check with your doctor if you have edema, kidney problems, or other medical conditions that affect your water intake.

Budget Stretcher #7: Use Fixed Meals. Research has shown that prepackaged meals (such as TV dinners) can significantly stretch your calorie budget. In one study, the dieters who had these portion-controlled meals lost 30 percent more weight than the others. The reason? With fixed meals, you know exactly how many calories you're getting. Apparently, our tendency to underestimate calories is not to be underestimated! So go ahead, and enjoy the convenience of a fixed meal several times a week.

Budget Stretcher #8: The Exercise Edge. My clients often ask me how important it is to incorporate exercise into their weight-control regime. I say, "Very." But I remind them, no exercise in the world can compare to the exercise of good *judgment* with your food choices!

The biggest budget stretcher is eating the right foods, but exercise gives you a crucial edge. That edge, however, may not be what people think it is. Exercise's greatest contribution is to success at weight control—because it gives focus and structure. It encourages the right *behaviors* for dieters . . . not just the calorie burn.

BUDGET BUSTERS

Budget busters are either high-calorie foods with very low thermogenic effect (like those high in fat and refined carbohydrates) or eating

Drink Tea for Weight Loss

We always have known that tea is delicious, refreshing, and thirst-quenching and in some cases may help reduce the risk of cancer.

You can now add it to the list of no-calorie foods that may help promote weight loss.

A recent study of more than 1,100 people in Taiwan, reported in *Obesity Research,* revealed that those people who drank at least one glass of black, green, or oolong tea per week for 10 years had 20 percent less body fat and 2 percent less abdominal fat than those who drank none. This was regardless of the amount of physical activity, food intake, and other lifestyle habits.

The researchers surmise that the tea may raise the metabolic rate while lowering the absorption of sugars and fat-producing molecules. This study is the most recent that relates tea to weight loss and adds evidence to what has up till now been a mixed bag of results. Multiple studies have suggested that tea promotes weight loss, whereas a few others have questioned its role. The best way to answer the question is once again to try it in your own life.

Chih-Hsing Wu, M.D., associate professor, Obesity Research Center, department of family medicine, National Chang Kung University Medical College, Tainu, Taiwan, was the leader of the study reported in *Obesity Research.*

behaviors that in various ways end up costing far too many calories.

Budget Buster #1: Eating Food "Just Because It's There." I would estimate that a good third to half of the calories my clients are consuming when they first see me are not from foods they particularly care about or would go out of their way to buy if they lived alone. Mostly they eat them because they happen to be around the house or office or right in front of them when they go out with other people. If it's in a bowl or basket within arm's reach, whatever it is, before long it's being nibbled on. I joke that their fingers have a "wait problem."

Snacks and other "nibble foods" are what make Americans most prone to lose control of their calorie budgets. In this country, it's estimated that almost *a quarter of all the calories consumed may be spent on snacking*—for some people, even more! Chips, nuts, cookies, candies, pretzels, regular sodas, and so on—you can find them almost anywhere in easy-to-eat-from bags and containers. *Snacks are "credit card foods": They make it easy to spend your calorie dollars without realizing the cost.* Each bite seems like a small, innocent amount, but the bill at the end of the month can make your jaw drop.

Oversize portions of high-caloric foods are also a particular problem in this and many other countries. The all-you-can-eat for $10.99 restaurant is a uniquely modern phenomenon. So is allowing our children to serve themselves whatever amount of high-calorie food they feel like heaping on their plates. This routine fosters feelings of deprivation when appropriate portions are served—an unhealthy attitude that's hard to break.

Years of observation have led me to form the E.A.T. principle—the **E**xpanding **A**ppetite **T**heorem: The appetite expands in direct proportion to the amount of food presented! *People are finishers.* People tend to finish what's on their plate. And the larger the plate, the more food we get served, so the more we eat. Even a larger *package*—the bag of chips, the box of cereal—makes us tend to eat more, independent of our hunger or its taste. This is just how humans behave, once again proving we are given to excess, not moderation, and we need strategy to control this tendency.

Even when people order healthful foods, they often ignore the quantity. So be alert for large portions or packages (especially of grains and other unmeasured nutritious foods).

Budget Buster #2: Eating High-Calorie Food Too Often or Indiscriminately. Some people prefer a great steak at a superb steak restaurant over a third-rate hamburger with Russian dressing with just as many calories. Others would rather have a superb 500-calorie dessert on a weekend. It's one thing to save up enough calories to allow yourself a treat from time to time. But it's quite another to eat it every day because it's on your kitchen counter or your restaurant's menu. Sometimes cutting out excesses such as these just requires a simple change in how you prepare or acquire food. Instead of baking a tray of cookies and finishing what your children don't eat, for example, just make one cupcake or muffin per child, so there's no excess. Strive to save your highest-calorie items for special restaurants where you get superb quality or for the special events that give joy to your life.

Budget Buster #3: Activity Eating. Some people are shocked to realize how many calories they spend on *activity eating:* eating just to be doing something when bored, anxious, or procrastinating; or eating associated with an activity, such as sitting in front of a TV or computer, talking on the phone, or reading. Many people say the weekends are the toughest. With all the unstructured free time in the afternoon or an evening home, people can get bored or a little antsy and may find themselves picking constantly all day or watching more TV and getting something to chew on during every commercial break.

And don't forget an insider tip: Keep the lights on bright, and you'll snack less. People tend to eat more in dark environments, research has shown. Ah yes, moviegoers!

Budget Buster #4: The 10-Minute Problem in Restaurants. Ten minutes is a very short time, but it can cost you more calories than the entire day if you're not careful. It can even cancel out the calorie benefit of hours spent in the gym. Winners at weight control realize that *the first and last 10 minutes in restaurants can cost more than the meal.* Good strategy is often needed in the first 10 minutes to resist the lure of too much alcohol or the breadbasket (which— did you ever notice?—no one seems to miss in a Japanese restaurant); and a salad dressing with more fat than a dessert. And in the *last* 10 minutes, there's the dessert question. What kind and what size portion does your budget allow?

So remember: The next time you want to reach for that roll or dessert menu—if you let the 10 minutes pass, it can save you hours in the gym. Your busy schedule will appreciate the effort!

Budget Buster #5: Hidden Calories. Are you overspending without realizing it? Most people realize that eating the wrong foods causes overspending, and if they cut them out, they notice a weight loss. But often after a period, the weight loss slows down radically or even stops, and my clients say they've "reached a plateau." *"Reaching a plateau" is typically an early warning sign of overspending.* I tell them they haven't reached a plateau, they've created one—usually by overlooking *hidden calories.*

Some calories hide in plain sight:

- **Too much of the right foods**—especially fruit, chicken, meat, and grains—can lead to calories you hadn't counted on.
- **The right foods served with the wrong ones**—the "sides" that come with a meal—can wipe out your calorie savings. An egg white omelet, say, that is served with home fries. The targeted eating strategy when ordering your entrée is to ask *What does it come with?* Don't be afraid of speaking up—you're the one paying good money for the meal, and your body is sharing the bill!

Other hidden calories are not so easy to detect:

- **The right foods prepared the wrong way** can bewilder dieters who often eat in restaurants and think they're ordering wisely but aren't losing weight. A classic example is calamari, which is very low in calories—except when cooked in butter or deep-fried! To avoid these hidden calories, always specify how you want your order prepared—even vegetables. Just saying one word—"steamed" or "poached" can save you 10 to 30 grams of fat on the vegetables alone. Steaming or poaching doesn't mean "no taste." If you ask them to steam the food with garlic and herbs or to poach it in wine or broth with herbs, most restaurants are happy to do so.
- **Salad dressing—a dessert on top of a salad.** Even the healthiest salad can cost an astonishing number of calories. A fine Italian salad with an olive-oil dressing can have as much fat as *three* quarter-pounders from McDonald's! Even though it may be "good" monounsaturated oil, from a weight loss point of view, fat is fat, and it's a weight-loss killer. Olive oil and Caesar salad dressings are the most common trip-ups—even the light versions. My clients often

order a shrimp or chicken Caesar thinking that the shrimp or chicken breast makes it a light meal, forgetting that some Caesar salad dressings can set you back as much as 30 grams of fat and many more calories than the chicken or shrimp themselves. Perhaps that's why Caesar had to always wear a toga! So always ask for "dressing on the side," and dip a fork into it instead of a spoon each time you want to add the dressing to your salad.

Budget Buster #6: Counting in Calories, Not Calorie Units. It may seem strange to say that counting calories busts your budget, but the truth is, many people may *count* in calories, but they *eat* in calorie *units*. It's not how many calories per serving that matters, but how many servings you typically eat. A few cashews may make up one serving, but most people don't stop with just a few. Or cereal—the average person pours into their breakfast bowl two to three times the amount given on the label as a single serving. And for someone with a history of finishing the whole bag of pretzels, the calories can end up three or more times the amount listed for a serving on the label. So it will serve you best to be honest about how many servings you really eat.

Budget Buster #7: Too Much Variety. As I've pointed out earlier, variety increases consumption, particularly at home. The more types of food you have around (especially nibble foods), the more you'll pick and eat and have food on your mind—and the hungrier you may feel. *The more foods in your pantry, the fewer clothes in your closet!* But when your taste buds encounter the same foods again and again, they get satisfied quicker. Too much variety keeps them curious and slower to signal "Enough." You go from one variety to the next, and your quantities and frequencies of eating increase. Limiting the types of food you buy and eat, for dieters, can have very big results!

Budget Buster #8: Trigger Foods. Trigger foods overpower your appetite's shut-off switch. They tend to *stimulate* rather than satisfy cravings and appetite, particularly foods made from white flour or sugar. Crunchy, bite-size foods such as nuts and candies are also hard to limit because you can quickly pop one after another mindlessly. When you surround yourself with such foods, you'll find that you're constantly thinking about them. "Always on my mind" in this case can mean "always on my behind."

Busting the Busters: The Secret Weapon

To correct for these budget busters, remember a simple technique that will cost you about 2 or 3 minutes a day but can save you *months* of fruitless, frustrated dieting or even failure: *Keep a food diary* (see page 162). Virtually all my clients who keep them find that they experience the same two results: (1) more awareness of hidden calories and therefore more weight loss and (2) a much higher level of success in *keeping* the weight off.

TARGETED EATING: HONORING YOUR PRIORITIES

Targeted eating is my strategy for avoiding or limiting the foods you care less about *so you can eat the foods you care more about or have them more often.*

Even if you extend your budget with calorienomic winners and exercise, your budget is still not infinite. First, you should spend it on food you need for good nutrition and energy. And the rest of your budget you can save for food you truly love (if you don't have a history of compulsively abusing it). For some, this might be a special dessert or even a holiday feast. Targeted eating gives you the freedom to enjoy these pleasures of your life. It builds up your calorie bank account. It also makes it easier to say no to high-calorie foods when you know you're saving the calories for something special you plan to enjoy soon.

So if you like to splurge on gourmet meals in a special restaurant or have a big dinner party coming up on the weekend, from Monday through Thursday eat light gourmet with our Phase A and B menus (see page 202 and page 245). Or if you know that you're going to a holiday dinner soon, save up calories by eating seafood or my Dr. G's World Famous Low-Calorie Zucchini/Eggplant Parmigiana (see page 222) for a few nights before and after.

Build up your savings by being *selective* about what you eat. The reason most people are overweight is that they *want* much more than they *need*. The goal of targeted eating is to pick what you want the *most,* so you can have what you *truly* need—the looks, the good health, the control, and the quality of life. Targeted eating also has the advantage of providing you with a safety zone in case you slip or fall from your diet.

Just as people save money for a rainy day, targeted eating puts calories in your body's savings account as a resource for special needs or treats—or if you should overeat. If you continue to balance your meals for good health and not spend too many calories on nonnutritious foods, targeted eating can put a great amount of pleasure in your diet.

BEING FOODSMART

Being foodSmart means picking foods that give you the *volume* you desire and let you eat more frequently. They provide high satiety but not high calories. This keeps your blood sugar stable and helps put an end to your cravings and hunger.

Winning at weight loss is never about losing the pleasure of food. Being foodSmart means finding great calorie bargains that offer great taste, satisfaction, and large volume with fewer calories. The foods on our eating plan and Taste Is King Awards list make it easy to be foodSmart.

High Volume, Low Calories

In 1994, when I wrote *Thin Tastes Better,* the advice of most weight counselors was to cut the food you're served in half and leave half on the plate. The diet approach I designed strongly rejected this behavior-modification approach to eating. All you have to do is go to a restaurant to realize this is not how real people behave. For most of my clients, there is no greater torture than sitting in a restaurant watching half your dinner grow cold as your friends finish theirs. And you still have to pay full price for half a meal! The "eat half, leave half" diet was contrary to the way people behave and a breeding ground for feeling deprived. People like volume!

Years after my book came out, Barbara Rolls, Ph.D., published an important, groundbreaking work in *Volumetrics,* which confirmed my approach scientifically. Her pioneering studies documented that *people want foods they can eat in large volume.* They will choose a large amount of food that's their second choice over a smaller portion of their first choice. Being foodSmart respects this basic human desire and gives you the volume you want without the extra calories. Instead of a tiny steak, order a nice, 2-pound lobster topped with pomodoro sauce or drizzled with a teaspoon of butter or steak sauce—for fewer calories! Or for dessert, instead of chocolate cake that sits there forlornly minus one sliver, have a delicious cappuccino with whipped cream. Or the enormous chocolate mousse pop I recommend in the food chapter (see page 175).

How to Save 40,000 Calories in 1 Month

Robb was a healthy but overweight man in his early thirties. A successful financial manager, he immediately understood the wisdom of calorienomics, and his expert budgeting skills and strategic mind made his diet program smooth and successful. I'd like to describe his typical eating day to show how painlessly you can lose significant weight by targeted eating and being foodSmart.

The first thing Robb realized was that the New York–style bagel he ate every morning was more than 400 calories, plus a couple hundred more for his butter or cream cheese topping. He had no trouble switching to a toasted English muffin (110 calories) with an egg (80 calories) and a spray of I Can't Believe It's Not Butter (zero calories). On some days, he had 2 tablespoons of low-fat cream cheese without the egg and a glass of fat-free milk. And when he had time for something more elaborate, he'd often make the egg white omelet from my gourmet recipes (fewer than 200 calories).

His usual lunch before had been a tuna wrap sandwich made with mayo and oil-packed tuna, which had several hundred calories and double-digit grams of fat. He switched to two sandwiches of ham and melted cheese with my recommended GG Scandinavian Bran Crispbread and light ham (two slices of ham and one slice of cheese per sandwich). This substantial, great-tasting, low-fat lunch gave him 12 grams of fiber and only 235 calories, so he also had one of my suggested soups for just 70 calories more. On other days, he'd enjoy three of my recommended light hot dogs (with plenty of mustard, which he loves) on a bed of sauerkraut (a mere 175 calories); or a delicious pastrami on rye made with the recommended beefsteak light rye bread (2 slices = 80 calories) and six slices of Hillshire Farms light pastrami (60 calories) and a pickle, topped with mustard, for a total of 150 calories. When he was in a hurry, he'd go to the drive-in window for a McDonald's Caesar salad (about 220 calories and 7 grams of fat) with half a pack of Newman's Own

Calorienomic Winners: The Favorites of My FoodSmart Clients

So what foods pass the thermogenic test and give you large volume so you never go hungry? What foods when made right have rich taste and texture, and people enjoy them because they're quick and easy to find and prepare? Here are the foodSmart winners most popular with my clients:

- **White-meat fish and seafood:** shrimp, crabmeat, lobster, scallops, cod, mussels, sole, orange roughy, flounder, skate, char, snapper
- **Egg whites:** egg white omelets, plain or with low-calorie cheese or foodSmart vegetables. Less desirable but still acceptable are egg substitutes or adding not more than one yolk.
- **High-calcium dairy foods:** low-fat/fat-free yogurt, milk, low-fat/fat-free cheese (cottage, ricotta, cream, American), protein shakes
- **Nonstarchy green and white vegetables:** broccoli, green beans, asparagus, artichokes, spinach, lettuce, cauliflower, zucchini, and cabbage. Vegetables such as these made without oil or butter are free under my program. And if you like "fried" vegetables, do them in a nonstick pan with a little chicken broth and olive oil spray or in the George Foreman grill. Vegetable burgers are also good if they're low in carbs.
- **Soups:** made from green and white vegetables and fat-free broth. They fill you up instantly.
- **High-fiber bran crackers** for safe, premeasured grain, for a fraction of the calories.

This is just a basic list of calorienomic winners. But wait until you see what we do with them in the food chapter, where you'll find as many gourmet entrées as you'll find in any gourmet restaurant in the world.

Light Balsamic Vinaigrette. He wisely avoided the packet of regular Caesar dressing—190 calories and 18 grams of fat!

At 4 o'clock, instead of cookies from the vending machine (240 calories, double-digit fat grams), he either had an apple (80 calories) with a light-cheese wedge (35 calories), or a chocolate parfait made with a cup of Total Yogurt, a tablespoon of Walden Farms Chocolate Dip, a few sliced strawberries, and a teaspoon of crunchy cereal for just more than 100 calories and no fat.

For his dinner salad, Robb decided he could forgo his usual creamy dressing of almost 300 calories for a teaspoon of olive oil and flavored balsamic vinegar for just about 40 calories. He had never liked bland steamed vegetables, but now instead of butter, he flavored them with garlic and herbs and the delicious, zero-calorie I Can't Believe It's Not Butter spray, saving hundreds of calories. And instead of his former main courses of pasta and cheese, or meat loaf, steak, or fried chicken—which average 700 to 1,000 calories—he now had shrimp with mushrooms and spinach, or grilled filet of sole in a mustard sauce, or my eggplant parmigiana (most of these meals average fewer than 300 calories). And on a night when he wanted dessert, instead of a fruit pie, he had my strawberry shortcake recipe, saving a few hundred calories more and multiple grams of fat.

At 9 P.M., he broke his habit of nibbling all night before bed by having a chocolate mousse pop for just 30 calories. And on those nights when he stayed up late and wanted a midnight snack, he enjoyed two scoops of my gourmet egg salad on two GG crispbreads for a little more than 100 calories.

There were some weeks when Robb grew so busy at work that he couldn't do his regular gym workout, but he continued to lose weight with variations of this menu.

At the end of the first month, Robb showed me a very professional-looking balance sheet, in which he had tabulated a savings of almost 40,000 calories compared with the month before!

After 90 days, he walked into my office looking great and smiling: He had lost more than 30 pounds! "It's terrific," he told me. "I'm never hungry anymore. I have tremendous energy. I have more than enough to eat, and the food is so good. And I'll be able to enjoy my wedding cake totally guilt-free!"

Robb's triumph can be anyone's. Calorienomics is not rocket science. It's a commonsense approach to weight loss that is uncommonly successful for both women and men. It's a triumph of being a selective gourmet and of knowing that weight loss does not mean giving up the pleasure of food.

Calorienomics helps us "do the numbers" for the life we want and the food control we need. As it trims our calorie budget, it also trims our figures and makes our dining richer.

Those who cannot remember the past are condemned to wear it.

The Tenth Thin Commandment:
Losing Weight Is Half the Job; Keeping It Off Is the Other Half

COMMANDMENT ESSENTIALS

- Remember to think historically, not just calorically.
- Keep in mind that even though you've lost the weight, you haven't lost your vulnerability.
- Stick to strategies and planning so you stay in control.
- Throw out all your larger-size clothing.
- Keep problem foods you have a history of abusing out of your house.
- Set a weight ceiling and defend it.
- Keep a photo of yourself at your heaviest weight.
- Keep a food diary.

HAVE YOU EVER HAD A REALLY bad toothache?

One thing it does is give you focus. All you can think of is relieving the pain. You'll even take off work for a day or change your entire schedule just to squeeze in a visit to your dentist. You'll endure a 6-inch needle's worth of Novocaine and hours in the dentist's chair—anything to stop the constant discomfort.

Starting a diet is like that. At first, you're super-motivated. Your weight has made you so uncomfortable that you'll stick with any diet. Mysterious powders, strange foods, and an odd eating schedule—you'll do anything to lose the source of your grief.

Warning: As the pounds fade, so does the pain and discomfort that gave you the focus to lose them! If you don't find a way to maintain your new habits, you might find yourself starting all over again.

This is the paradox of weight loss: It may be the only area of human behavior where success doesn't seem to breed success. Whether it's a business executive closing a big deal or a runner winning a race, their victories inspire them to want more. What is the reason that so many of the winners at losing weight fail to stay in the winner's circle?

They all want to keep the weight off. Hunger and deprivation are clearly not at issue—most maintenance diets offer more calories and much greater variety. It's not a knowledge problem—dieters don't suddenly forget what foods they were eating to keep their calories and carbohydrates low and lose weight. They don't lose sight of the foods they were eating. If that were the case, they could easily refresh their memories by returning to the diet plan or diet book they were following.

Still, there must be a reason why so many people who succeed at losing weight fail at the critical juncture of keeping the weight off. How do we best explain this phenomenon?

What is the winning path through this critical juncture: *weight gain or weight maintain?*

WHY DO SO MANY PEOPLE FLUNK MAINTENANCE?

When you're losing weight, encouragement is ubiquitous. You have an automatic barometer—the scale—to chart your progress and friends and family members to shower you with compliments or an occasional pat on the back. It's easy to stay structured and focused.

But then you hit your desired weight, and the well runs dry. The compliments come less frequently. The scale stays in a holding pattern. *On maintenance, it's no longer about the scale dropping but about the scale not going up.* Now, the very real, but less tangible concept of living your life in control of food is the goal.

When someone is losing weight, their body is getting lighter, their clothes are loosening up, and their appearance is improving. The goal is within reach. You think this would be something worth protecting. But as I have shared with you in the pages of this book, human behavior is often not about logic, but rather *psychologic*— the logic of the psyche. Sometimes, we don't follow even the most carefully crafted script.

We're all vulnerable to the normal human tendency to let down our guard when we no longer feel threatened. The human psyche is programmed to forget pain. Our minds distance us from unpleasant experiences with the passage of time. It's part of our psychological survival mechanism. So how do you survive on maintenance when the pain and discomfort that inspired weight is a thing of the past?

When it comes to weight control, we move away from the very pain and discomfort that motivated us to start dieting. Under these conditions, it's easy to be lulled into thinking that once you lose the weight, your problems are solved. *In truth, it's only by employing successful strategy and winning at maintenance that you can ever really solve the problem.*

The classic diet model suggests that there is a beginning and an end—one that ends with weight loss. *In truth, there may be a beginning and an end to weight loss, but never to weight control.* All the studies show that the winners at weight control don't just lose weight. They make real, tangible changes in their thinking. And the *greatest* change occurs in their approach to maintenance. This is why the word "diet" comes from the Greek word *dietos,* which means "way of living." This is the true meaning of diet and dieting.

Some who flunk maintenance lose the structure of their eating. And what is a diet but a *structured* way of eating? As many people reach their target weight, the gloves come off, and all foods become green lights with only a single admonition: all foods in moderation.

This would be great if we were inclined toward temperance. However, people are not given to moderation but to excess. I would argue that the statement "all foods in moderation" is more of an idealistic than realistic statement about human behavior.

In fact, the philosophy of "all foods in moderation" sets people up to overconsume and flies in the face of research that suggests that too much variety actually encourages overeating. As Tara Parker Pope observed in a recent edition of the *Wall Street Journal,* "Variety excites the appetite . . . and stimulates consumption." Some studies have shown that people who choose from a variety of foods will eat 50 percent more than those given a single food.

Also, when something tastes great, the tendency is not to moderate but to finish. This is the pleasure principle of the human psyche.

I'm not refuting the "all foods in moderation" mindset just to be argumentive. I simply want to explain why you may have failed before on maintenance.

A few years ago, the *New York Times* reviewed my work and found that almost 50 percent of the clients they surveyed had kept off 20 to 100 pounds for at least 5 years on maintenance—and I didn't preselect the clients they interviewed. They stated that this success rate stood in marked contrast to the success rate in the field for a 5-year period, which they reported that many experts estimate at around 10 percent. When one considers two additional factors, this finding becomes all the more remarkable. Many of these people had not seen me in several years, yet they were still successful. They didn't need to come back for additional visits because they were employing the strategies on their own—techniques you have learned about in this book. The strategies had become for them, as for many of my clients, automatic and easy. Through them, they had found lasting success.

Secondly, the people who came to me from throughout the tri-state region of New York, the country, and the world have a terrible track record with dieting. Typically, they have tried everything and failed everything. I'm a "court of last resort" for the "terminally dieting." Most of my clients have been to the top weight-control specialists and programs at universities, teaching hospitals, and spas. A very large number of them are privileged to live a life where they select only the best of the best for health care without regard to cost or insurance reimbursement. And yet they have not found success through years and decades of trying with weight programs—and the best trainers for exercise. Yet, using the strategies of *The Thin Commandments Diet,* years of failure have ended with victory over their weight problems. I am honored and humbled to have been a part of this victory, for truly they deserve it.

I know of no other program where so many people have kept off so much weight for so long. If you follow the strategies in this book, you too will reach the winners' circle on maintenance.

Once the weight goes, the Thin Commandments still apply. And for maintenance, in particular, never forget the second one: Think Historically, Not Just Calorically. Forgetting this commandment is perhaps the *greatest* reason why so many who get an "A" on weight loss flunk maintenance. Many maintainers shift back into caloric thinking alone. The weight is gone, and they wonder, "What's wrong with just a taste of this or that food?"

Well, there's nothing wrong—if they have a history of only being a taster with this or that food. But if they have a history of abusing that food, taking a taste reactivates the craving memory. If you have to fight cravings and hunger every day, how can you expect to control your weight?

WINNING AT MAINTENANCE

The motivation for losing weight is pain and discomfort with your weight. So after the weight evaporates, you need a *shift* in motivation. In fact, a wholesale change in thinking is needed to make the great leap from weight *loss* to weight *control*.

Winners at maintenance let the process be the goal. To live your life in control of food is the process *and* the new goal of maintenance. If you don't have power over food, you'll never be in command of your weight. This is the essence of maintenance!

Successful dieters know they've lost their weight, not their *vulnerability*. Just because you lost 20 or 30 pounds, your taste buds haven't changed. You still have the same number of fat cells. You still have the same personality. *Most important, you still have the same history with the foods that made you heavy!*

Throughout this book, I've used the word *paradox* to clarify a statement that may seem counterintuitive. Perhaps the greatest paradox of all is what I call the paradox of maintenance: *The only way to lose the problem is to realize you never lose the vulnerability.*

Losing weight does not mean you're less susceptible to the aroma, taste, or texture of certain foods. If you were in the habit of overeating crunchy, salty, or sweet-tasting foods before, you'll still be vulnerable to them on maintenance. Whatever started the ball rolling before will start it rolling again. Imagine what can happen if you add

20 different types of foods to your maintenance diet that share these characteristics. You'll be adding a lot of stimulation—and temptation.

Feeling above temptation is a red flag on maintenance. Because the moment you believe you're secure, you run the risk of thinking, "Why do I need strategies and planning?" That's when the enemy of thin rushes in: complacency. Only by knowing you're being tempted can you resist temptation. *Sometimes the greatest temptation of all is the temptation to become complacent.*

The winners understand that the weight is a symptom of being out of control with certain foods—and certain behaviors. However, it's not the only cause of their problem. The real cause is the food, behaviors—and the thinking. Remember, losing weight is not the equivalent of earning a college degree—something you do once and then forget about. Many people believe that losing weight is solving the problem. In truth, it's only half the job.

Keeping it off is the other half.

The Story of Janet

One of my clients, Janet, a busy executive who had kept weight off for many years, noticed that she was returning to an old habit of stopping for a candy bar on the way home from her office. Before too long, she was back craving sugar and abusing sweets.

What Janet didn't realize was that eating a candy bar on an empty stomach when her blood sugar was low—she often skipped lunch and/or her afternoon snack—was causing her appetite to spiral out of control for the rest of the night.

If Janet had remembered one of the lessons of the Third Commandment, The Problem May Be in the Food, Not in You, then she would have known that the chemical byproducts created when carbohydrates, such as candy bars, are burned as fuel stimulate a group of nerve cells in her brain to produce neuropeptide-Y, a chemical messenger that made her hungry for even more carbohydrates and sent her appetite into overdrive.

I pointed out to Janet that eating a candy bar at the end of the business day was the perfect setup for an evening of appetite and sugar cravings. By starting with this candy bar when

Maintenance: The Importance of Thinking Historically

Like a child let loose in a toy store, people on maintenance often avail themselves of all the foods the world has to offer. Suddenly, the world is their oyster.

There's just one problem. If they could limit themselves to just a few oysters, they wouldn't have needed a diet to begin with!

To succeed on maintenance, they need fresh guidelines and a new structure based on their own inimitable experience with food. This last point is vital. Otherwise, the person might think the new code was being imposed on them from the outside. But when they know the principle is culled from their own history and behavior—not from some generic eating plan—they feel compelled to honor it.

One of the most critical lessons I've ever learned for success on maintenance is this: *Those who honor their history keep it off; those who violate their history fail.*

her blood sugar was low and her body was craving carbohydrates, she was throwing a match into gasoline. Janet would have been much better off treating herself to a protein meal at one of New York's five-star restaurants after a long day because fine food was not her "issue"—but candy was!

If Janet had one of the protein-rich, low-fat yogurts I recommend or a shrimp cocktail, she would have put an abrupt end to her daily blood sugar roller-coaster ride.

This news was a revelation to Janet. She told me, "Now, I finally realize that it's not about me—that I'm not lacking motivation or willpower. It's the food I'm choosing that's causing me to spiral out of control again."

Janet's years of success at weight control did not change her vulnerability to the truth that eating behavior habituates very quickly or that she is a sugar-sensitive person with a long history of losing control with sweets.

No matter how intelligent you are or how secure you feel, you're no match for the force that is your body's physiological response to a food. *This fact doesn't change just because you're on maintenance.*

Thinking historically, not just calorically, is the new guiding principle.

When a client asks, "Can I have some peanuts, a candy bar, or a piece of bread from the breadbasket now that I'm ready for maintenance?" I ask him a simple question in return. "What is your history with this food or this type of food?" No one has a problem answering this question.

Knowing my clients' histories with food or groups of food gave me insight into their behavior and the ability to identify potential pitfalls and forks in the road. It was like clearing the field of landmines before the tanks rolled through.

So when one of my clients, a prominent film executive legendary for his negotiating skills with the toughest Hollywood agents, was contemplating a return to breadbaskets, I asked, "When in your life did you ever negotiate with a breadbasket and win?" Needless to say, he never returned to breadbaskets. And now for the first time, after decades of failure at weight loss, he is succeeding.

By confronting my client with the truth of his own history, he realized that it was easier to live without a destructive habit and that doing so would increase the likelihood of lasting success at weight control. The insight ended his habit of failing at maintenance.

Also, cutting out just one food that was costing him thousands of calories a month gave him freedom to enjoy thousands of other foods—without the fear of gaining weight.

My client's story points out another great truth about maintenance. *True deprivation starts when you return to foods you have a history of abusing because they're certain to rob you of success at weight control.*

10 Tips for Keeping the Weight Off

Here are 9 critical behaviors and 1 additional shift in thinking that make up the 10 most important things to do on maintenance. The first 4 behaviors characterize all my winners. The 6 additional behaviors describe most of my clients. And while I believe that all 10 are important, the first 4 are critical for success.

SPECIAL ALERT: The single most important thing you can do to keep weight off for a lifetime is so important I've changed the format of the text to indelibly etch it into your psyche.

1. **Wear form-fitting or tight clothes!** When you reach maintenance, you should have one size, and one size only, of clothing. I've found that *nothing* sounds the warning siren faster or motivates people to act with greater haste than when their clothing gets too tight!

   Think about what motivated you to start your diet. If you're like many of my clients, you were uncomfortable with your clothing (or you couldn't fit into it) and appearance. When you have a little extra trouble buttoning a pair of jeans or find it necessary to add an extra notch to your belt, it reawakens the original motivation. When you have only one size, you have no choice but to stay trim. If you save larger sizes, you are making it easy—too easy—to just switch to a larger size instead of acting to correct any errors.

   Also, if you don't plan to be heavy again, why save the larger sizes? *When you reach maintenance, throw out the larger sizes—immediately!*

   Knowing that you have only one size of clothing adds another powerful incentive to maintain your weight: *economics!* How many of us can afford to buy a whole new wardrobe—especially one in a larger size? Your wallet gives you extra incentive to guard your weight loss.

   Before people ever respond to the clarion call to health, they listen to the cry of their clothing getting too tight. I'd have a nearly empty office if I tried to motivate people to stay on maintenance on the basis of health alone.

   Your wardrobe is the most powerful deterrent I know of against sliding once more into out-of-control eating. It signals your commitment never to be heavy again. That's why I insist that all maintenance clients discard all clothes that no longer fit, with one exception: I ask them to save the outfit that's their largest size (preferably one they disliked ever having to wear) as an eternal reminder.

2. **Keep problem foods you have a history of abusing out of your home.** *Almost all* the women and a very large percentage of the men I have worked with who regained weight started the slide in their own homes. The slide often began with a

food they had a history of abusing but had avoided while they were losing weight.

Remember the study by researchers at the National Weight Control Registry that found that two out of three people who lose weight and keep it off keep problem foods out of their house? Although that food might not tempt you at this moment, I can't urge you strongly enough to remove it from your home or at least keep it permanently out of your sight. Remember, you're always vulnerable to the foods that have tripped you up in the past—even on maintenance. Eventually, people tend to return to their old favorites if they are continually available. On maintenance, even more than weight loss, availability stimulates craving—even if it doesn't happen immediately. Along with keeping only one size of clothes in your house, it's critically important to keep problem foods out of your home.

3. **Set a weight ceiling, and defend it.** Pick a number—typically about 3 pounds for women, 5 pounds for men—and don't let your weight go above it—ever. No matter what happens, don't let yourself off the hook. Draw a line in the sand. If you see your weight going up, return to my A list eating plan for several days, and as the weight starts to move down, you can add selections from my B list. When the weight is back down, you can return to maintenance eating (my C list). Most of my clients expect increases in weight on weekends because of higher-calorie maintenance meals at home and out. Monday is typically the "high number" day of the week, but by Friday, they bring the weight back down to their goal weight, via Phase A and B eating.

4. **Weigh yourself every day.** Your bathroom scale can't weigh your behavior. However, it will tell you when you gain a pound or two. If you step on the scale the morning after a big meal at a restaurant or special event, your weight could be up. Don't be alarmed. If it's water weight, it will dissipate in 24 to 48 hours. You should expect slight variations during the week, especially after maintenance meals.

If it's real weight (3 or more pounds that remain over a

period of several weeks), that should be a warning to you to take immediate action.

If you find it a bit maddening to follow the daily fluctuations of the scale even though you are eating properly, pick three days of the week on which you will always weigh yourself (for example, Monday, Wednesday, and Friday).

5. **Weigh yourself on the Maintenance New Scale,** a nearly foolproof way to predict the scale of tomorrow (see page 162).

6. **Exercise.** It gives you structure and control. It gets you thinking about calorie burn and health consciousness and directs you away from obsessing about food. It's been shown that dieters who exercise regularly succeed the longest at keeping weight off. A study of more than 32,000 dieters by *Consumer Reports* magazine found that "regular exercise was the number one successful weight-loss maintenance strategy" of more than 81 percent of the long-term maintainers. In second place, at 74 percent, was the related strategy of increasing activity in daily routines. Also, as your body becomes lighter, it burns fewer calories. Exercise helps expand your calorie budget by burning the higher-caloric foods of maintenance.

And remember: Exercise generates endorphins, increases energy, and elevates mood.

Exercise provides you with a healthy outlet for stress. These effects help you follow through on your commitments, especially to control your weight. And as an outlet for stress, exercise shortcuts mood eating. It's the perfect alternative to keep your moods out of your foods.

7. **Keep a photo of yourself at your heaviest weight.** For added emphasis, place it next to a picture at your lightest weight. Many of my clients put the photo in a place where they feel most vulnerable—the refrigerator door or kitchen counter, for example. Others elect to carry the photo in their wallet or purse.

Some of you may find it upsetting to stare constantly at a picture of yourself at your heaviest weight. Instead, carry a picture of what you look like at your lightest weight. You may find it motivates you even more to protect your accomplishments.

The Maintenance New Scale

In the first chapter, I spoke about the importance of weighing yourself on the New Scale for Dieting to guarantee that you'd lose weight. I've modified the first chapter New Scale to reflect the new guidelines and thinking necessary for maintenance success.

This simple, 10-question quiz reviews some of the basic skills and attitudes that increase your likelihood of success at weight control. Take this quiz once a week after you reach maintenance. If you answer "yes" to four of the questions, it's an early warning that you're slipping into bad habits. If you answer "yes" to five or more questions, you're in danger of regaining the weight—even if your scale hasn't started to rise yet. If you see that you're slipping into old ways of thinking or violating your history in some way, just admit it. Evaluate what caused you to slip, the situation, and where it might have occurred. See what you can learn from your mistakes so they won't happen again. Remember, slips should teach you, not defeat you.

1. Am I eating any foods that I have a consistent history of abusing?
2. Am I getting sloppy about my behavioral strategies and failing to plan?
3. Am I eating too much of the right foods?
4. Am I nibbling again on whatever foods are around?
5. Am I being negligent about weighing myself regularly and guarding my weight ceiling?
6. Am I keeping problem foods in my house?
7. Am I skipping meals or snacks or going longer than 4 hours without eating?
8. Are my clothes tight?
9. Am I allowing my moods to dictate my foods?
10. Am I skipping exercising frequently during the week?

When it comes to weight control, a picture is truly worth a thousand words.

8. **Keep a food diary.** I'd like you to keep a diary for at least the first 90 days on maintenance. I ask my own clients to keep a diary for a full year. I want them to be certain they can manage the entire cycle of the year, with its holidays, vacations,

special events, birthdays, summer versus winter eating, and so on. Since the same events and seasons come up year after year, once you get through the first year, you should be well prepared for the coming ones. After the first year, I frequently ask some clients to continue to keep a food diary or to keep a record of any "error" such as eating problem foods or excessive quantities of caloric foods.

A diary will serve as a daily reminder of the extras and/or negative eating habits. Writing out your meals and snacks a day in advance will help structure your thinking and help you steer clear of potential trip-ups.

9. **Give yourself clear boundaries.** Boundaries are a strong structure for your eating behavior. A major study of the winners found that 88 percent limited some type or classes of food. Another 45 percent limited the quantities of the foods they ate. Remember, if you don't have a good history of limiting a particular food, avoid it.

   I help my clients establish clear boundaries and control their calorie budget with the lighter menus of Phases A and B of my eating plan from Monday through Friday, saving their maintenance meals or higher-calorie foods for weekends and special events. This clear boundary helps build an infrastructure of positive behaviors and smart eating habits that becomes automatic after a few weeks.

   Most of my winners reinforce their boundaries with the techniques of Box It In and Box It Out. Many decide to Box Out a certain category or type of food. For some, it's baked goods, especially breadbaskets. Others avoid sweet baked goods (but may indulge in another type of sweet, such as a chocolate mousse). I want to emphasize again: They don't do this to make their lives difficult or to deprive themselves of something they want. They do it to make it *easier* to succeed at weight control—which is something they want more.

10. **Go beyond the food reward system.** My winners enjoy the pleasure of fine food. Many of them dine regularly at fine restaurants. However, they've evolved beyond the childhood programming that views food as a reward or a treat.

They understand that no matter how beautiful a food looks or how enticing its aroma, if it's a food they have a history of abusing, it's no reward at all.

Some of my clients reward themselves with new clothes. Others enjoy a trip to a spa, a new necklace, or a weekend getaway with friends.

These are material rewards. *A far more meaningful reward occurs each morning when they look in the mirror and see a trim body.* There's no greater reward you can give yourself than to live the vision you have for your own life.

RECORDING YOUR OWN INTERNAL VOICE

When I sat down to write this book, I had a goal in mind to share with you every technique I've used to promote success at weight control. Since many studies have shown that staying focused is a key to weight loss, I make a tape for each of my maintenance clients.

The tapes were designed to reinforce the goals of maintenance and to facilitate the new strategies into their day-to-day living—and to make certain they don't forget the mistakes and lessons of the past. As I've said before, the only way to get permanent weight loss is through permanent changes in your behavior and eating habits.

My clients find that one of the best ways to guard these changes is to listen to their maintenance tapes. Some listen to their tapes every few weeks. Others listen every day or whenever they need a friendly reminder.

The sample script I've provided you with (see page 166) is similar to the one that's kept my clients focused and successful.

On your tape, you may want to address problems or challenging situations that might be coming up in your life. However, always end your tape on a positive note by speaking to your strengths. Remind yourself that you have the smarts, not the food. Also, make a note to yourself that if you're upset or disappointed, that "it's not about the food." Every time you eat in response to life's disappointments, you give up power over your own destiny. Happy, sad, rich, or poor—it's still better being thin. Or should I say "staying thin."

The 10 Biggest Maintenance Busters

Successful weight control extends beyond knowing what strategies work best. It's also about learning to appreciate the forces that can chip away at your resolve and long-term success.

I've identified the top 10 maintenance busters. They may not lead to failure immediately, but over time, they erode your control and healthy new eating habits.

1. **Skipping meals.** Special bulletin: A new study indicates that the number one behavior that leads people to gain weight is skipping meals!

   Perhaps the greatest maintenance mistake is skipping meals or going too long without eating. This habit, which some people engage in to lose weight, will cause your blood sugar to dip and can increase your appetite and cravings.

   Some people are trained to believe that if they eat three meals a day, they'll be fine. You can eat three meals and still go too long without eating because there are too many hours in between meals and snacks. Some people decide to skip lunch or, worse, breakfast. Others neglect to have the required late-afternoon snack. On maintenance, missing this snack is the equivalent of skipping a meal.

   If you have lunch at noon and don't eat dinner until 7, you've gone too long without eating (remember Janet's story on page 156). This will make it more likely that you'll overeat at dinner or fall prey to night-eating syndrome.

2. **Nibbling.** There are few things that can undo your control and the structure of your eating habits faster than mindlessly picking or nibbling on foods you have a history of abusing or picking on whatever foods you happen to encounter in the course of a day.

   Worse, most people don't count what they nibble and pick on toward their calorie budget. Nibbling is like a cancer that insidiously eats away at your calorie budget.

   Once you grant yourself permission to eat whatever's in your environment, everything becomes fair game. Slowly, the calories start going up while your control starts heading south.

Sample Tape: Maintenance

These are some of the major themes I use on my clients' tapes, which I've found to be the most powerful and help produce the greatest success on maintenance. Not all these statements may apply to you, so pick the ones that resonate the most, or create new ones just for your lifestyle—and your history!

- Losing weight is half the job; keeping it off, the other half.
- "My new goal is one day at a time, to live my life in control with food and to avoid any foods and behaviors that weaken my control (list any particular negative foods or behaviors). There is no food I can't have. There are foods I may choose not to have because they don't work for me."

- "I have lost my weight but not my vulnerability, so I need to stay focused."
- "I didn't come this far to take orders from a piece of food."
- Think historically, not just calorically.
- Remind yourself that this way of living is an infant in your life and needs nurturing.
- Remind yourself of the trigger foods and behaviors that each time you returned to, you gained back your weight. If you have trigger foods you have Boxed Out, remind yourself of them and the mantra "I don't take the first little taste; I don't begin; I don't have any problems." Reiterate again for your psyche: "The first taste is not about the calories but the crav-

Nibbling becomes a habit that can quickly become as addictive as any drug.

The three meals and two or three snacks on my eating plan give you structure. Nibbling destroys that structure. Remember, finger control is the essence of weight control—unless you're nibbling one of the "free foods" such as green and white vegetables (which I will explain in the diet chapter). Once you go back to nibbling on whatever food(s) happen to be lying around, you sacrifice eating structure.

On maintenance, it's critical to keep clear boundaries with nibble foods. Don't deviate unless it's a planned indulgence with a fixed amount of food. And avoid eating with your fingers unless you choose a low-calorie food from my eating

ings. I don't reactivate cravings."

- Remind yourself of challenging situations that might be coming up or any problems you may be having with food or your eating behavior.
- "This work is not about dieting but about the quality of my life."
- "This work is not about deprivation, but liberation: liberation from a lifetime of weight problems and failing again and again with my weight on maintenance."
- "If I choose to avoid a certain food, it's not that I can't have it. I avoid it because it doesn't work for me."
- "If I'm not planning, I'm planning to fail."
- "I need to stay focused, otherwise, I'll be focused on why I'm heavy and miserable. One way or the other, this will be on my mind each day, but now I'm on the winning side, and I plan to stay there."
- "I deserve to be trim. I deserve to succeed at this. I deserve to be in control of my life with food."
- Complacency is the enemy of thin—stay focused.
- "I think like a winner—to be trim and successful is my greatest treat, goodie, and dessert."
- "I have life smarts; a piece of food doesn't."
- "I'm finally free to live the vision I have for my own body."
- "Finally, I have a new taste: the taste of thin, the taste of success. This is worth protecting!"

plan, such as the shrimp, fruit, crudités, or my own recommended bran crackers.

3. **Eating too much of the right foods.** After weeks or months on a diet, people are generally more aware of the types of foods they're eating. However, they're often not as aware of the *quantity* of the foods they're eating.

Many of my clients have gotten into trouble eating too much of the "right foods" such as chicken, beef, and even fruit—particularly when they're nibbling from bowls of cut-up fruit or bowls of grapes and cherries. Some ate too much because it was an "allowed" food, and they assumed that portion size didn't matter. Others got into hot water when they ate what they thought was only a single serving, when it was actually two or three times that amount. (This typically happens in restaurants, especially with pasta dishes.) To correct for this, just have pasta as an appetizer.

There's a tendency on maintenance to let quantity fly under the radar. But it can contribute thousands of extra calories to your diet. When a client tells me she's following the protocol, but still gaining weight, I often suspect that the culprit is too much of the right foods.

4. **Reactivating cravings.** There's a popular misconception in the field of weight control that the way to eliminate a craving is to eat the food you're longing. For some who don't have a history of compulsive eating or have never abused that food, this may be true. For the rest of us, eating foods we have a long history of abusing (such as trigger foods) does not satisfy cravings—it fuels them.

If you think that just tasting a food you've decided to Box Out is not *calorically significant,* you're right. However, from a control point of view, you're dead wrong. Any time you stir up interest or reactivate cravings in a food you've elected to avoid, you give your psyche a green light. Once you tell yourself it's okay to have a little, you're inviting temptation and overconsumption. You start looking for the food again, you start thinking about it, and you start noticing it more, or worse, you start buying it and keeping it around your home— even though it's a food you have a non-history of being a "taster" with and a long history of excessively abusing.

5. **Letting the supplies of healthy food run out.** Even my most well-intentioned maintenance clients have run into problems because they overlooked a simple but key ingredient for success. You can't construct a building without the right tools. Similarly, you'll never succeed at maintenance if you don't have enough of the right foods.

After some of my clients get to the goal, they stop buying the foods that contributed to their success. They become careless about stocking their homes with the right foods. It's not that they don't like these foods or intended to stop eating

THE TENTH THIN COMMANDMENT

them. Since the goal has been achieved, buying the right, or should I say "calorienomic winners," no longer seems paramount. They soon start eating the higher-caloric foods that are around the house for others. Another danger is that they stop stocking their ThinPack, and they end up eating whatever foods happen to be around in meeting rooms or when they travel. Before too long, this becomes the new habit.

6. **The add-on effect.** On maintenance, I often see people continually adding new foods to their diet without attempting to balance their calorienomic checkbooks. Even if you choose healthy foods such as whole wheat bread, brown rice, and fruit, you need to balance your budget by subtracting or substituting for the extra foods you add.

Simply because you're excluding or limiting foods you have a history of abusing doesn't mean you can add one new food after another to your diet. When a maintenance client asks if she can add a new food, and I see that her weight is stable, I remind her that her body doesn't need any extra calories. So, if she wants to add a new food(s) today, I ask her what she's willing to subtract from her calorie budget tomorrow. Or, I'll tell her to add a couple of extra days of light eating to her diet. On maintenance, people tend to practice "one-way mathematics"—only addition. They forget about subtraction, substitution, or division. Watch for this maintenance buster; it often eludes notice.

7. **Returning to mood eating.** You can lose all the weight you want, but if you run to food the next time you're upset, you're jeopardizing your chances for lasting success on maintenance.

Sometimes when people are losing weight, they refuse to eat—even if something bothers them (demonstrating that they clearly have the power to control mood eating), since they are determined to lose pounds each week. Once they've lost the weight, it's easy for them to slip back into the old habit of eating every time they're anxious or annoyed. Yet, they will be a lot more upset if they start losing control and regaining the weight.

Feeling in control in your own life can be a bulletproof

vest against the slings and arrows of life's annoyances and misfortunes.

Sometimes success on maintenance is not about your foods, but your moods. Stay alert!

8. **Creep syndrome.** People don't go to bed trim and wake up heavy. Weight gain is a slow, subtle process that often goes undetected. Most people don't get too alarmed if they gain back a pound or two. Or, they rationalize. You might hear, "It's only 1 or 2 pounds, so it's not a big deal." Before too long, those 2 pounds have morphed into 3, and that same person says, "It's just 3 pounds." And the 3 becomes 5, 8, and then 10.

This is why I insist that you set a weight ceiling, guard it, and make no excuses. And if that number starts to go up, take action! Before you even realize it, those 5 or 6 pounds can turn into 15 or even 20.

9. **Failing to plan.** Planning is about protectiveness. When you start a diet, the desire to lose the weight and look and feel better pushes you to plan. After you lose the weight, you may believe there's nothing left to protect and, therefore, no urgent need to plan.

You may stop carrying your ThinPack, or find yourself going to restaurants hungry, or going food shopping when you're most vulnerable.

Often, failing to plan goes undetected. It can take the form of something as benign as sitting near an open bowl of nuts or not moving the breadbasket out of arm's reach. Even these subtle planning blunders can have a *dramatic* effect on your cravings over time—and your success at maintenance.

Losing weight does not reduce the need for planning. Actually, planning makes things easier because it guards your success. It helps you avoid pitfalls and establish boundaries.

Remember, if you fail to plan, you're planning to fail.

10. **Tomorrowisms.** "I'll do it tomorrow. Just not now." Does this sound familiar? It's the promise of someone who sees that they're gaining weight back but puts off going back on their diet.

It's also a reflection of what I like to call *maintenance resistance*. Once someone grows accustomed to the greater variety on maintenance, they often resist returning to lighter food even if their weight starts going up.

If you know that you're prone to maintenance resistance, it's important to act quickly. When it's just a few pounds, you can take off these pounds typically in a week or 10 days. So even if you're resistant, you don't have to push yourself for too long. The longer you delay, the more your weight goes up, the longer it will take to get it off, and the more maintenance resistance increases. Also, your weight is increasing because you're eating too many calories and returning to negative eating habits. If you're returning to old habits, it's important to end them quickly, not to keep reinforcing them through delay.

To help you do this, write out a day or week's eating plan in advance. Tell yourself, "If I stick to this, I'll lose X number of pounds." Also, try ridding your home of any foods that might be tempting you to eat incorrectly.

If you're still having trouble or find you can't do it alone, enlist a friend who also wants to lose weight, and give each other mutual support, join a weight program, or contact an online support group, such as ediet.com. Many of my clients also find that going to a spa for a few days or a week gets them away from trigger foods and unhealthy eating habits and jump-starts their motivation. I often send my clients to quality spas such as Canyon Ranch to recharge.

Don't be a passive observer when you see negative behavior.

Remember, the more you say "tomorrow," the more you'll weigh tomorrow.

These 10 maintenance busters don't require much interpretation. However, the insouciant, devil-may-care attitude of some is more subtle and creates a fertile breeding ground for problems. When you realize that *the process is the goal*—to live your life in control of food—that your maintenance journey is just beginning, I believe you'll appreciate the need to protect and not to "test yourself" or the boundaries.

When a client says to me, "I just wanted to test myself," I smile and remind him that the reason he's sitting in my office is that he already tried to test himself—and flunked. And if that attitude persists, he'll be a perfect candidate for flunking maintenance.

THE ONLY COMPLIMENT YOU'LL EVER NEED TO HEAR

There is only one way to achieve permanent weight loss, and that is to make a lasting change in your eating habits. This is the truth. It would be far easier for me to say to each of you, "All foods in moderation." And that's what I would wish for all people. But as I've said throughout this chapter, that's not the behavior of all people. The statement "all foods in moderation" is only for those who are given to moderation and whose history bears this out. For the rest of us, strategy comes first.

If you follow the strategies in this commandment, whether you choose my diet or any other weight program, one thing is certain: You'll do maintenance in a new way and get a fresh result—success. Most important, you'll hear the compliment most dieters never hear—"You've kept it off!"

Then you'll know you've not only lost the weight, *you've also lost the problem.*

PART II

THE THIN
COMMANDMENTS
DIET

The ABC Eating Plan

I call my eating plan the ABC Eating Plan because it makes weight loss as easy as ABC. The weight loss is quick and easy, and the guidelines are easy to follow. All the foods are readily available at supermarkets, health food stores, and gourmet food stores, or you can order them by telephone or via the Internet from the resource section at the end of this chapter.

There's an A-list of foods and recipes for those who want to lose weight quickly and safely. *The A-list is a synergistic combination of foods that literally turbocharges your body's capacity to lose weight.* These foods make up my 10-Day TurboCharge Diet.

There's a B-list of foods for those who want to stay on the program for longer than 10 days or have more than 10 pounds to lose. It offers greater variety than the A-list and some higher-caloric foods and recipes. The weight loss in this phase will be somewhat slower.

Finally, there's a C-list of recipes and foods for when you've lost your weight and you're ready for maintenance—or any time you want to temporarily stop your weight loss. It offers even greater variety and higher-caloric choices—in addition to the foods of the A- and B-lists—for your maintenance lifestyle. The maintenance section also recognizes that there are some dieters who are very concerned about having too many choices and less structure on maintenance. They prefer to do maintenance with an eating plan similar to their weight loss program, so I also provide guidelines for this group.

There's a unique bonus with the ABC Eating Plan. It offers five-star dining with my unique food selections and foodSmart recipes, yet it gives the most rapid, safe weight loss possible. I believe that any dieter would give that an A.

WHY IS THIS THE BEST DIET FOR YOUR WEIGHT LOSS?

Typically, diet books become part of the popular culture and then, inexorably, fade into obscurity. However, it seems that as soon as a book fades from our collective consciousness, another pops up to take its place. This year alone, scores of new diet books will hit the shelves of bookstores around the country, each promising a new and better way to help you lose weight.

So, in this increasingly crowded marketplace, where there are literally thousands of diets and diet books to choose from, how do you decide? *As you read these words, you may find yourself asking, What makes a diet the best diet for me?*

If you're reading this book, you've probably tried your fair share of diets. You may know of or have used a dozen strategies for counting calories and shedding excess pounds—perhaps only to fail time and time again. You may have lost weight on your diet of choice but were often left feeling hungry, frustrated, and, most important, deprived.

After working nearly 30 years in the field of weight management, I know that picking the right diet is not a matter of serendipity. *To succeed at weight control, you must choose a way of eating that is livable so you can step off the diet merry-go-round and lose the weight you want without hunger or deprivation.*

In the last three decades in weight management, I've asked thousands of people to describe their "ideal diet." Their answers seldom vary.

- The diet must provide safe, rapid weight loss.
- Taste is king—the foods must taste great and look great.
- It has to leave me feeling satisfied, not hungry or deprived.
- It has to allow me to eat more and still weigh less.
- It has to make me look and feel better.
- It has to be healthy and provide superior nutrition.
- It must provide options for those who want variety and also provide the option of a structure to accommodate those who don't want to make too many decisions about food and don't want variety.
- It has to have clear guidelines so I don't eat too much.

- It should maintain my energy level or give me more energy.
- It has to be uncomplicated and filled with foods that are easy to prepare.
- It has to fit to my normal lifestyle, which includes work, going to special events, restaurants, parties, and eating on the run.

What if I handed you a diet that not only met these criteria but also gave back structure and control and honored your food history?

Throughout my career, I've experimented with countless diets. The one I'm about to share with you produces the best weight loss, gives the most volume, and prevents craving and hunger, all while offering a dazzling array of low-calorie, great-tasting foods. I've said before that if I were to give an eleventh commandment, it would be this: It's not about deprivation, but substitution. The foods and menus in this chapter will prove that axiom.

Putting this eating plan together involved more than jotting down a few words on a page. There are decades of thought behind it. Anyone can tell you what you need to eat. But wouldn't you rather know how to live free of the cravings and feelings of deprivation that are the constant companions of most dieters? This is the end result of smart strategy and the right type of diet.

For many of my clients, this eating plan has produced *more* than successful weight loss. By knowing the right foods and having the right strategies, they've brought an end to the painful chapter of failing at weight loss.

WHY IS THIS DIET UNLIKE ANY OTHER DIET?

Time and time again, so many of my clients, particularly women, complained they couldn't lose more than a few pounds on other diets. Further weight loss became nonexistent or a constant struggle. How is it that this diet has made all the difference?

I believe it's my diet's synergistic combination of foods that literally turbocharges your body's capacity to lose weight that makes all the difference. Many diets look at how food affects the body and weight loss. Others center on counting calories, grams of fat, and carbohydrates. This diet goes beyond those parameters to fulfill the promise of calorienomics by giving you foods that

- Offer safe and rapid weight loss
- Allow you to keep taste and texture without the calories
- Increase volume while decreasing calories
- Promote satiety—so you feel full and are never hungry
- Respect your need for structure
- Meet your nutritional needs
- Eliminate the negative effects that many diets have on your behavior in the form of cravings, hunger, small quantities, lack of energy, and bland foods that stir feelings of deprivation

The ABC Eating Plan includes foods that support the behavioral strategies you need to help you lose weight. It respects and honors your individual food history by excluding foods that could lead to out-of-control eating. *Most important, this eating plan avoids the foods that are most often abused and that sabotage the weight loss of many determined dieters.*

The selection of foods on my menus and shopping lists come from my own observations and from countless hours spent sifting through thousands of pages of scientific studies, many of which, I believe, will influence diets in decades to come.

In the Ninth Commandment, Treat Your Calories Like Dollars, I spoke of the power of certain foods to promote greater weight loss over foods of equal calories. This part of the book will further explore the weight-loss benefits of three special foods— and one food group with a magic mineral—that will help you jump-start your weight loss and keep it off for a lifetime. First, you'll learn why I call seafood the "Concorde to Thin" and why it's one of the best choices for *rapid* weight loss, satiety, superior nutrition, and looking younger and living longer. You'll also find out about the weight-control benefits of the spice cinnamon and how it regulates the hunger hormone insulin and may help you in losing weight—and even lowering your bad cholesterol. Yet it has no calories, and it tastes great. I've also found cinnamon helpful in keeping sugar cravings at bay.

Next, I'll explain why high-fiber foods are so effective at diminishing appetite and why GG Scandinavian Bran Crispbread may be the crown jewel of this group. It's such a great appetite suppressant that I call it the "hunger killer."

Finally, you'll discover that by simply eating foods rich in the mineral calcium, specifically dairy foods, you might be able to increase your weight loss by 70 percent. Through this synergistic combination of foods, along with the recommended amount of water and suggested teas, you'll be able to eat more while taking in fewer calories—as well as lose more weight. *Who said a calorie is just a calorie?*

Everything You Need to Lose Weight— Quickly and Easily

The ABC Eating Plan lists the best foods to help you lose weight. Then it offers suggestions and guidelines to keep that weight off permanently. *This eating plan also avoids one of the most common pitfalls for people losing weight, which is a sense of deprivation that comes from feeling they're missing out on the pleasure of food.*

This eating plan is literally bursting with dozens of five-star dining recipes ordinarily available at only the finest gourmet food stores and most exclusive restaurants. Now, you can have them at your home— inexpensively and quickly. Inside, you'll discover true five-star dining in the form of luscious desserts, gourmet entrées, and scrumptious snacks lovingly created especially for you by Chef Miriam—the first female cook at the Four Seasons, one of New York's most celebrated restaurants. I'll also treat you to a sneak peak at the menu of Solar Harvest, a unique new eatery set to open shortly in Los Angeles, featuring "premium, quick casual dining." You'll even get some of the personal recipes for meals I serve in my own home, such as zucchini/eggplant parmigiana, cinnamon French toast, shrimp scampi, egg salad, and light pizza. *This plan is proof that losing weight doesn't involve giving up the pleasure of food or missing out on the fun of fine dining.*

This chapter was designed as a minibook within a book. In addition to menus filled with great-tasting gourmet recipes, you'll get six simple strategies for effortlessly navigating the supermarket aisles and an extensive list of delicious, low-calorie brand-name foods. Resources, on page 302, lists contact information for many of the recommended brands. Stocking your pantry and refrigerator has never been so easy.

As a special bonus, you'll get a list of more than 100 "best of the best" light foods on the market that taste as good, if not *better* than their higher-calorie counterparts. *Without these foods, my clients would never have lost so much weight without deprivation!* This list (page 294) will quickly simplify your food shopping. You'll immediately know what to look for the next time you go to the market. And you'll put an end to sorting through hundreds of "low-calorie" and "low-carbohydrate" pretenders that disappoint your taste buds.

This chapter also gives you sound, practical guidelines for handling planned splurges, a way to reduce facial bloat in just 10 days, and advice on what to do if you've reached a weight-loss plateau. Most of all, it's a plan that makes it easy for you to join the ranks of the winners at weight control.

What are you waiting for?

FOUR FOODS THAT GIVE YOU AN UPPER HAND AT WEIGHT LOSS

Have you ever heard someone talk about a great poker player? Typically, they'll say something to the effect of "That guy just can't lose. He's probably got an ace up his sleeve." In other words, he's got an edge—an advantage that virtually guarantees him the winning hand.

I believe that those of you embarking on the ABC Eating Plan also have an edge. But instead of having just one ace up your sleeve like a star poker player, you have four. That's right. You have four aces that just might help you reach your target weight and keep that weight off for a lifetime.

As I mentioned in the introduction to this chapter, the entire ABC Eating Plan emphasizes three foods and one food group with a magic mineral, all of which allow you to keep the taste without the calories. Now, I'll explain to you what they are and why they just might put you, as they've put thousands of my clients, on the short path to rapid, safe weight loss.

Why Seafood Is the "Concorde to Thin"

Think about the last meal you ate. Did it leave you satisfied, or did you find yourself thinking about eating or reaching for more food a short time later? Many things influence how much you eat, and now research is showing that satiety may be one of the most important factors. Simply, satiety is the feeling of fullness or satisfaction that occurs when your stomach and intestine signals your brain that you've had enough. If you want to shed pounds quickly while reducing a few inches from your waistline, it's not just the amount but also the type of food you choose that may matter the most.

For as long as I can remember, I've championed seafood, especially shrimp and fish, and called it the "Concorde to Thin" a decade ago in my book *Thin Tastes Better.* Now, it appears that scientific evidence may prove me right. Seafood has always been one of the very best sources of low-calorie, vitamin-rich, nutrient-dense protein and may also be one of the best choices if you're looking to fill up faster, control hunger, and *ultimately* lose weight at an optimal rate—even if you've been unable to lose weight on other diets.

Fish gets the highest marks on the "Satiety Index," a way of measuring how full people feel during a 2-hour period after eating 240 calories worth of food, developed by obesity expert Susanne Holt, Ph.D. The more protein, fiber, or water a food has, the more it satisfies.

On Dr. Holt's index, *fish came in second overall to boiled potatoes as the most satisfying food per calorie and was the only protein source at the top of the list.* Since most varieties of finfish and shellfish provide between 100 to 200 calories per 3½ ounces, based on the Satiety Index, they're among the best choices if you're looking to fill up and feel satisfied. Bulky high-fiber foods, such as fruits, grains, and vegetables, also rate high. But they can't compare to fish. Needless to say, many baked goods, including cookies and cakes, finish near the bottom, because 240 calories worth is often a small portion of these foods.

Based on the 240-calorie ceiling, you could have 7 ounces of shrimp, 21 medium-size scallops, 9 ounces of boiled lobster, 5½ ounces of salmon, or 2½ pounds of mussels (in the shell). Assuming, of course, you could eat that much at one sitting!

Dr. Holt's findings support what I've taught for years—that a key to controlling weight is to eat foods that have fewer calories per ounce, so you ultimately leave the table satisfied without blowing your calorie budget.

Virend K. Somers, M.D., Ph.D., a professor of medicine in the division of cardiovascular disease and hypertension at the Mayo

Clinic, and a man whose scientific work I admire greatly, has a theory about why fish may be one of the best foods for weight loss.

Dr. Somers says that fish may influence your body's production of *leptin,* a hormone manufactured by your fat cells and secreted by your fat tissue. In people, leptin is a satiety factor and acts on the hypothalamus, the part of your brain that regulates appetite. The level of leptin circulating in your bloodstream, says Dr. Somers, is often directly proportional to the amount of body fat, or adipose tissue, you have. For example, women generally have more body fat than men and tend to manufacture more leptin. Researchers at Rockefeller University found that the amount of leptin correlates to how much fat is stored in the body. Higher leptin levels are found in people with more fat and reduced levels in those who dieted.

Dr. Somers believes that fish "may change the relationship between leptin and body fat, *making the body more sensitive to leptin's message of satiety.*" Perhaps this is why fish is the only protein at the top of the Satiety Index.

This heightened sensitivity to leptin's satiety message may have critical applications to helping you lose weight without ever feeling hungry. Earlier in this book, I discussed how the protein *neuropeptide Y*—described in one study as "the most powerful appetite stimulant yet discovered"—increases food intake—especially for carbohydrates—and stimulates secretion of insulin and cortisol, which can lead to fat accumulation. Leptin may counteract the effects of neuropeptide Y. Leptin may also offset the effects of anandamide, another powerful feeding stimulant, and promote the synthesis of α-MSH, an appetite suppressant. The result: lower food intake. A Purdue University study found that leptin may inhibit the synthesis of fat in fat cells and increase the burning of fat in muscle cells.

One of the nation's leading nutritional researchers, Michael Zemel, Ph.D., has observed that leptin "decreases appetite and increases metabolism." *When it comes to having a meal, fish may be the ultimate calorienomic food for decreasing appetite, giving large volume and low calories, and turbocharging your body's capacity to lose weight. In fact, fish may stand alone in the entire world of food in offering these benefits for your success at weight loss.*

The Benefits of Fish

Fish offers so many positives for dieters that it's hard to list them all in one sitting. However, the following are a few you might want to know about:

- Fish is nutrient dense, meaning it offers large amounts of protein and significant minerals and vitamins without a lot of calories and saturated fat.
- The protein in fish is easily digested.
- Fish contains small amounts of fat (most types contain less than 5 percent). Even higher fat varieties, such as salmon, still have less than 15 percent, which is lower than most cuts of meat. Fish is also lower in saturated fat than many other protein sources, such as chicken and turkey.
- Fresh fish, not canned, is generally low in sodium. Most varieties of fish contain 60 to 100 milligrams per 3½ ounces. Excess salt can contribute to bloat and increase your blood pressure.
- Fish leaves you feeling more satisfied after a meal.
- Fish is loaded with unsaturated fatty acids, called omega-3 fatty acids. Omega-3 fatty acids are one of two types of essential fatty acid—the other being omega-6 fatty acids— that our bodies can't manufacture on their own and can only be derived from food. Some studies have shown that omega-3 fatty acids may improve our cells' sensitivity to insulin, thereby reducing our chances of developing excess body fat. These same fatty acids may also increase thermogenesis, so that more of the calories from your food are burned up during digestion instead of being stored.

Cinnamon—A Simple Way to Spice Up Weight Loss

In your wildest dreams, could you conjure up a delicious, zero-calorie food that may help you control your hunger, lose weight, and possibly even encourage the development of your lean muscle mass? If you thought, even for a moment, that such a food existed, would you frantically search the Internet or scour the globe to find it? Fortunately, you may not have to resort to such extreme measures. More than likely, you'll locate this food during a 5-minute visit to your local supermarket. How's that for quick and easy?

If you've eaten a baked apple or piece of French toast in the past week, you may have enjoyed cinnamon and didn't even realize it. Many of you know that cinnamon tastes great on a variety of foods, but what you may *not* know is that cinnamon may be one of the best foods for weight loss. It turns out that consuming just ½ teaspoon of ground cinnamon daily may help control your hunger, keep your waistline in check, and even gain more lean muscle. Does this all sound too good to be true? Well, it isn't, at least according to Richard A. Anderson, Ph.D., lead scientist at the Beltsville Human Nutrition Research Center in Maryland and one of the country's foremost authorities on the effects of food on human metabolism.

To start, says Dr. Anderson, cinnamon improves insulin activity in fat cells. When you eat a meal, your pancreas releases insulin (a protein), which prompts your cells to take in the glucose (sugar) floating in your bloodstream. Fat cells, notes Dr. Anderson, utilize sugar. So the more excess sugar you have, the more fuel your fat cells have. In other words, your fat cells start getting fatter. Cinnamon makes your cells use insulin more efficiently, thereby increasing sugar metabolism—a process by which your cells convert blood sugar to energy. By limiting the amount of sugar in your blood, you're depriving your fat cells of their sole source of food. Dr. Anderson's latest research shows that cinnamon cuts blood-sugar levels by 20 to 30 percent.

To control your weight, keep your blood-sugar levels stable. As Dr. Anderson so adroitly noted, "Whenever there's a problem with someone's weight, there's often a problem with his or her sugar."

Cinnamon may aid weight management by helping control hunger. Simple sugars, such as the type found in cookies and white bread, require relatively little time to digest and cause a rapid rise in your blood-glucose levels. When this happens, your pancreas produces a corresponding amount of insulin, so your blood-sugar levels don't go through the roof. This large, rapid insulin response often causes your blood sugar to fall too low just a short time after the cookie or bread is finished. Before long, you may find you're hungry for something else. Typically, you'll reach for more cookies or a similar food to get your blood sugar back up. "Since cinnamon helps control the amount of insulin your body needs, it ultimately controls satiety. If you're not hungry all the time, you'll take in fewer calories," says Dr. Anderson.

In my own work, I have used cinnamon very effectively to help control sugar cravings and found it to be particularly helpful for lessening PMS cravings. Many of my clients have used cinnamon as a creative strategic tool to put a quick end to carbohydrate bingeing with baked goods and bread products. *It is a powerful tool for your error correction and containment in the arsenal of the strategies you have learned in this book.*

Most significant, cinnamon may help you lose weight by increasing your body's production of lean muscle mass. Because cinnamon helps increase sugar metabolism, it frees up insulin to perform one of its other important jobs: lean muscle development. Insulin controls the uptake of amino acids (the building blocks of protein) into muscles, which increases the synthesis of muscle protein. "When insulin doesn't have to spend a lot of time controlling your blood-sugar levels, it can spend more time converting amino acids into protein, which leads to increased lean body mass," says Dr. Anderson. By adding cinnamon to your diet, it may be possible to lose weight without decreasing lean muscle mass.

A central goal of my eating plan is weight control and fat loss. In which case, a good long-term solution is one that improves insulin sensitivity, controls hunger, and promotes the development of lean muscle. Cinnamon just might do all three.

Dr. Anderson's findings confirm what I've observed firsthand in my work—that cinnamon augments flavor while simultaneously enhancing satiety. Frequently, foods that improve taste stimulate cravings. Cinnamon seems to do the opposite. I've also found that cinnamon helps turn off sugar cravings and restores blood-sugar levels after too much carbohydrate bingeing.

As an added bonus for your health, cinnamon may lower total cholesterol, bad cholesterol, and triglycerides anywhere from 13 to 30 percent. That's comparable to the benefits seen with statin drugs. Dr. Anderson says that boiling one cinnamon stick in a cup of water to make coffee or tea will give you the same effect as ½ tablespoon of ground cinnamon.

Volumize with Fiber

Eat more fiber. You've probably heard that advice before. But do know why you should eat more fiber?

Fiber has many functions, but it is probably best known for its ability to relieve and prevent constipation. But what you may not know is that high-fiber foods, especially my GG Scandinavian Bran

Crispbread and the green and white vegetables on the ABC Eating Plan, offer three big benefits for people looking to lose weight, as leading nutrition writer Jane Brody recently observed in her weekly column in the *New York Times*. "They hold water in the gut and take longer to digest, and some of their calories are eliminated unabsorbed. In other words, they can fill you up before they fill you out."

To start, your body absorbs fewer calories from foods high in fiber because your digestive enzymes can't break fiber down, which means that your body can't absorb it. This is why high-fiber foods, provided they are low in fat, also tend to be low in calories.

Since your body absorbs so little fiber, many researchers now say the grams of fiber in a food can be subtracted from the total grams of carbohydrates in the food. This results in a net carb count, meaning you count only those carbohydrates that have a tangible effect on your blood sugar. For example, a cup of spinach has 4 grams of carbohydrates but also 3 grams of fiber, so its effective carb count is 1. To be "carb smart" means to choose foods that have a favorable ratio to fiber and to avoid the ones that don't (such as regular bagels, processed breads, pasta).

Many high-fiber food choices allow you to engage in an activity I have described as *volumizing. Simply put, volumizing allows you to eat large amounts of food while taking in fewer calories.* Certain fiber-rich foods provide a lot of volume, or size, for the calories, so you can eat more of them without packing on extra weight from the calories.

Equally important, high-fiber foods tend to make a meal feel larger (partially because they bulk up after they enter your stomach) and remain longer in your stomach, which may help you stay full longer. Since it can also take up to 24 hours for high-fiber foods to pass through your digestive tract, they can help control your appetite—and calorie intake—for up to a day.

Similarly, fiber also slows down nutrient absorption after a meal, thereby controlling your blood sugar and reducing the amount of insulin your body needs. Large volumes of food activate stretch receptors in your stomach, which then send a signal to your brain that you feel full. To activate these receptors faster, you're better off with foods that provide large portions with low calories, since the number of calories you consume has far less impact on satiety than volume. For example, half a cup of brown rice equals 115 calories; but a 100-calorie serving of fiber-rich, garlic-roasted broccoli equals

OptiCarb Eating

As I said earlier in this book, *opticarbs* are foods that promote weight loss by accelerating your body's ability to lose weight while also tending to eliminate the hunger and cravings that sabotage success on so many diets.

The ABC Eating Plan draws on cutting-edge research to include a select group of foods that work synergistically to optimize the body's ability to lose weight, even in those most resistant to weight loss.

This group of foods is further enhanced by what I call the opticarbs—a unique group of low-carbohydrate foods that promote *success* at weight control by:

1. Enhancing your body's ability to lose weight so that you lose significantly more weight on a diet that includes these carb foods over a diet with other carb foods of equal calories.
2. Controlling hunger and cravings, especially for the "bad carbs"—high-glycemic carbohydrate foods that cause fast, dramatic spikes in your blood sugar, which may, in turn, contribute to weight gain.
3. Providing you with generous volume and superior nutrition for relatively few calories.

These "smart-carb" foods include:

* High-calcium dairy products, especially yogurt, high-calcium dairy shakes, and low-fat/nonfat cheese and milk
* Green and white, low-starch vegetables, such as cucumber, spinach, broccoli, cabbage, asparagus, mushrooms, celery, salad greens, and green peppers, which give volume and fiber for appetite control and satiety, plus super nutrition. These vegetables are so low in calories and carbs that you can include them as free foods.
* GG Scandinavian Bran Crispbread. The GG is the only grain that gives your body 0.0 "net" carbs, while supplying more fiber and fewer calories (and fewer carbs) per ounce than other grains.
* Grapefruit—the only fruit with carbs that has been demonstrated to accelerate the body's capacity to lose weight.

It is this mosaic of foods that I call opticarb eating. These are the carbs that promote success at weight loss. That's why I say ABC Eating is opticarb eating. It gives you the carbs without the consequences!

4 cups. Which do you think is going to fill up you up faster?

Finally, many fiber-rich foods, such as broccoli and asparagus, require more time to chew, which gives your body more time to register when you're no longer hungry, so you're less likely to overeat.

Some of you reading this may be curious why I've made no mention of grains, which are by all known standards an excellent source of fiber. While I do like some grains—specifically the GG Scandinavian Bran Crispbread—and include them in my eating plan, I've found that they may not be the best choice for dieters. For one, grains do not provide the one thing you want most: volume at low calories (which you can see from the previous example of brown rice compared with broccoli). Indeed, if the goal is to put more food on your plate, why limit yourself to tiny portions of brown rice and whole-

Lose Your Carb Face in 10 Days

Shakespeare said: "God has given you one face, and you make yourself another."

The face tells all. For most of us, the part of our bodies that shows the first signs of weight gain and bloat or weight loss is the face. While many of my clients complain that they can't fit into their clothes or grouse about wanting to lose their belly fat, what really shows up first is weight gain in their faces. If you've ever looked closely at a person who has put on a significant amount of weight or has binged on carbohydrates, his face often looks puffy and distended. This is what some of us who work in the field of weight management call the "carb face."

There are a lot of things that can cause you to acquire a carb face. As luck would have it, some of the foods we love the most are the worst thing for our appearance. In particular, refined carbohydrates, especially those found in baked goods, some crackers, pretzels, breads, and pasta, may cause your body to retain fluid. In fact, for every gram of carbohydrates you take in, your body tends to retain 3 to 5 grams of water. Many of these products also contain excess amounts of salt, which may compound facial bloat. Most refined carbohydrates are also high on the glycemic index, a scale that rates foods according to their impact on blood-sugar levels. High-glycemic foods are digested quickly and flood your bloodstream with glucose.

wheat pasta, when you can have large portions of foods such as spinach sautéed with garlic and ginger, two steamed artichokes topped with a tablespoon of Walden Farms calorie-free salad dressing, or Dr. G's Light Pizza on two GGs for fewer calories—and fewer carbohydrates?

Portion control is another problem with grains. I've found that people tend to overeat grain-based foods—even healthy choices like brown rice and other grains, especially when served in restaurants or in unmeasured quantities. I don't mean to disparage grain products. Provided they're not fried or prepared in oil and you don't have a history of abusing them, they can be helpful. But in terms of calories per ounce, you'll do much better with green vegetables. Or get your fill of grains, as my clients do, from the GG Scandinavian Bran Crispbread, which gives volume, crunch, satiety, and low calories.

Whenever that much sugar is present in your bloodstream, your body responds by releasing insulin to bring your blood-sugar levels back to normal. When sugar increases insulin levels in the body, more calories and fat are stored.

The good news about following the eating plan is that it not only reduces your weight and cuts inches from your waist, but it can also close the door on facial bloat. If you do the 10-Day TurboCharge Diet of my A-List, with its abundance of low-carbohydrate foods, many of which are rich in skin-friendly DMAE, you'll see a great improvement in your bloated carb face. Just as the face is the first to show weight gain, the reverse is also true. It's also the first part of your body to show

weight loss when you follow the right type of diet. Remember to drink plenty of water to facilitate the process.

I've often said that your clothing is the first line of defense to keep you from gaining weight. You might want to think of your face as the second battalion. If you've ever had a night of carbohydrate bingeing, you may notice the next day that your face looks puffy. Reducing facial bloat will accentuate the appearance of your weight loss, making it appear as though the pounds are literally melting away. My clients tell me that the first thing they notice after going on the 10-Day TurboCharge Diet is a reduction in their facial bloat. It immediately makes them look trimmer.

Lose Up to 70 Percent More Weight with Calcium

There's an expression, "Don't cry over spilled milk." Well, if you knew what dairy products could do to turbocharge your weight loss, you just might shed a tear or two the next time a glass of milk hits the floor. And this isn't the latest fad; it's real science. At least according to one of America's premier nutrition researchers, Michael Zemel, Ph.D.,

What to Do if You're Doing Everything Right But Still Not Losing Weight

It doesn't happen very often. But every once in a while, a client will tell me that he's honoring his history, using good strategy, following the eating plan—and still not losing weight. Sometimes, it's the seemingly innocuous amounts of food you unconsciously put in your mouth throughout the day that, over time, add the extra pounds. For instance:

- A mother might help herself to a few chips or the last few bites of a sandwich, or eat several spoonfuls of pasta her toddler couldn't finish. It may seem hardly worth the effort to refrigerate such a small amount, and why let it go to waste? That is, of course, until you realize that those three or four spoonfuls could add up to an extra 150 calories.
- You've just come to the end of a box of cereal and notice that a few ounces have spilled into the bottom of the box. Why, you might think, let it go to waste or spend the effort returning it to the cupboard? Well, those few tablespoons could add a few hundred calories to your breakfast.
- You go food shopping and help yourself to a small sample of cheese and crackers. No problem, right? Except that cheese and crackers could end up costing you 150 to 200 calories (a 1-inch cube of regular Cheddar cheese contains about 110 calories).
- You're whipping up a batch of chocolate chip cookies for your daughter's soccer team and find there are a "few" spoonfuls left at the bottom of the mixing bowl. One spoonful equals a single, medium-size cookie, and you just ate four (300 calories).
- You're sitting at a bar, waiting to meet a friend for dinner and decide

chairman of the nutrition department at the University of Tennessee.

In a 6-month study, Dr. Zemel discovered that people whose diet consisted of 3 to 3½ servings of low-fat dairy, or 1,200 to 1,600 milligrams of dietary intake from dairy foods, lost 11 percent of their total body weight. *Most significant, they lost a lot of body fat, especially around the waist area. Dr. Zemel concluded that adding three servings of low-fat dairy a day can help you lose up to 70 percent more weight,*

to help yourself to a "small" handful of peanuts before she arrives. That handful of nuts could be costing you anywhere from 200 to 300 calories.

- You go to Starbucks each day for a jumbo coffee, forgetting that adding extra milk, or worse, cream may have just upped the calorie count of your drink 25 to 30 percent.
- You're dining at your favorite restaurant, and the waiter brings you a dressed salad with a *few* croutons or pieces of tostini on top. A ½ cup of garlic croutons has 86 calories and 3.5 grams of fat. The salad dressing may have a few hundred calories.

Does any of this sound familiar? As you can see, these little bites of food can add many calories to your diet and possibly several inches to your waistline. What's even worse, they can easily start a daily pattern of "little extras." Fortu-nately, it's not too difficult to avoid these mystery calories. The following are a few of my favorite strategies to help tilt the scale back in your favor.

- **Keep a journal or diary.** Writing down the foods you eat is a good way to avoid those little nibbles that add extra calories. In your diary, circle any foods made with sauces, oils, or those containing extra quantities. You might cut back on the nibbling because you simply get tired of writing down everything you eat.
- **Carry your ThinPack.** Take a few healthy, low-calorie snacks, such as a few GG crackers or an apple, with you so you won't have to give in to higher-calorie temptations.
- **Never cook or go into food situations hungry.** You're more likely to overeat or give in to a food you have a history of abusing.

increase body fat loss by 64 percent, and help you lose 47 percent more belly fat. Yes, you read that correctly.

I can't tell you how many of my clients, especially women, complain about not having a flat stomach or not fitting into their clothes. Perhaps the most familiar refrain I hear in my practice is, "I can't get rid of my stomach bulge."

Most of us do not get enough calcium in our diets. And if you are among those getting the lowest levels of calcium—255 milligrams a day as opposed to the recommended 1,000 milligrams— you are 84 percent more likely to be overweight than if you are among those getting the highest level—1,346 milligrams per day. As Dr. Zemel noted in his excellent book, *The Calcium Key,* "Wouldn't you love to be 84 percent thinner just by eating more calcium-rich foods every day?"

When calcium levels are not kept optimal, observes Dr. Zemel, your body releases a hormone called *calcitriol,* which, in part, *controls* how fat cells work. If you don't get enough calcium in your diet, calcitriol is released, and your fat cells get fatter—and you gain more weight! *High-calcium diets suppress calcitriol levels and may speed up weight loss.*

If you're thinking of adding more calcium to your diet, some of you may be wondering if calcium supplements are as efficient at lighting a fuse under excess weight and stored fat as dairy foods. While supplements do help—the subjects in Dr. Zemel's study who took an 800-milligram calcium supplement along with 400 to 500 milligrams of dietary calcium daily lost 7.5 percent of their total weight without reducing calories—they don't provide nearly the same boost as dairy products. "Dairy products contain a number of bioactive compounds—similar, we believe, to the phytonutrients found in plants— that exert a much stronger effect on fat cells than supplements," says Dr. Zemel. One of these compounds, L-leucine—an essential amino acid—is especially interesting because it helps lower elevated blood-sugar levels and may make fat cells behave more efficiently.

Years ago, I noticed that my clients who added calcium-rich foods to their diet lost more than those who did not. Yogurt is the top calcium-rich food. A cup of plain or vanilla yogurt can have up to 490 milligrams—almost half the recommended daily requirement. Other calcium-rich dairy foods include milk (1 cup has 390) and cottage cheese (½ cup has 75).

Other Points to Keep in Mind

In addition to your weight loss slowing or reaching a plateau, you should also keep the following points in mind regarding your overall health when starting a new weight loss program.

- **If you have low blood pressure.** If you have low blood pressure, losing weight may cause your pressure to fall farther, and you may feel faint (especially if you don't drink enough water or you go too long without eating). When dieting, it's a good idea to drink generous amounts of water, and you may even want to include some higher-salt foods such as pickles and certain commercial soups, such as Imagine Organic Free Range Chicken Broth (11 ounces for 5 calories), to keep your blood pressure stable. In general, if you have a history of low blood pressure, hypoglycemia, kidney stones, gall bladder problems, low potassium, heart problems, or diabetes, you should lose weight only under the guidance of your physician.
- **If you change your diet.** In a small number of people, switching from a diet containing a lot of refined carbohydrates to a lower-carbohydrate diet causes a mild "withdrawal effect." In the first day or two, they may feel weak or experience headaches. If this happens to you, drink plenty of water and take an aspirin or Advil (unless you're allergic to those medications), and be certain to eat every 3 to 4 hours so your blood sugar stabilizes.
- **If you're taking medications.** If you're taking medications for diabetes, high blood pressure, or other conditions, your prescription may need to be adjusted as you lose weight. Always speak with your doctor or pharmacist if you have any concerns, but *never* adjust medication on your own.
- **If you experience leg cramps.** Low potassium or inadequate fluid intake may cause you to experience leg cramps. If you suffer from leg cramps, it's important that you check with your physician about taking extra potassium. A small banana, two to four slices of cantaloupe, or a glass of tomato juice will help bring your potassium levels back to normal. Your doctor can run a blood test to check your potassium levels. And if you suffer from kidney, gallbladder, or heart disease, you should only diet under the supervision of a physician.

THE ABC EATING PLAN

If you're reading these words, you probably have a clear idea about the new standard for weight loss and weight control. You know that your unique food history is the "North Star" to help guide you safely through the world of high-calorie temptations and trigger foods. You're familiar with the strategies for Boxing It In and Boxing It Out. You've learned how to rid your vocabulary of self-defeating "food baby talk" and replace it with a new script. And you've overcome the feeling that following an eating plan that keeps you trim equals a lifetime of deprivation. You realize that structure gives control. And you know that the goal of this eating plan is not just to lose weight but to permanently change behavior patterns that have doomed your past attempts at dieting.

So now that you've absorbed the lessons of *The Thin Commandments Diet,* you're ready for one of the most enjoyable parts of this book: the ABC Eating Plan.

Before embarking on this diet, many clients will say, "I know what foods to avoid and what foods are best for weight loss. But what should I be eating every day, and what will make it simple as possible?"

So now I'll share with you the answer I share with them: You can eat a lot, and you can eat well. You can eat any food on the plan—*provided you don't have a long history of abusing it.* But remember that some foods have more calories than others and can stop or slow down your weight loss.

As I've already mentioned, the ABC Eating Plan is separated into three parts. The first part of the diet—the A-list foods——which I call the 10-Day TurboCharge Diet, includes foods that produce the quickest weight loss and don't take a lot of time and effort to prepare. The second part of the diet—the B-list foods, which I call the Continuing Plan—offers menu choices for more moderate, sustained weight loss and is recommended for those who want to stay on a diet for more than 10 days. And finally, in the last part of the diet—the C-list foods—or Maintenance Phase, I've included additional higher-calorie, gourmet choices for variety and guidelines to help you sustain the weight you lost in the first two phases of the diet, all while enjoying your normal lifestyle. The menu options in this phase of the eating plan still respect your history and need for structure, which is essential for long-term success.

Anywhere in the ABC Eating Plan that you see two amounts or portion/serving sizes for a given food, the higher amount always applies to men and the lower amount to women. This rule applies to all three parts of the diet and extends to all foods I recommend, including gourmet meals, recipes, snacks, desserts, drinks, and minimeals.

A-LIST FOODS:
THE 10-DAY TURBOCHARGE DIET

Often, when people begin a weight program, their eating habits have been sloppy and lacked structure and focus. A well-designed, well-organized eating plan—one with clearly defined guidelines, instructions, menus, and foods—will help rein in even the most chaotic eaters almost immediately. This is why giving you too many food choices to start may cause you to feel overwhelmed and lose structure. So the items I've included here are lower in calories (for fast weight loss) and a little more limited in terms of the variety of foods offered on the second and third parts of the eating plan. Once you have your structure firmly entrenched, then you can broaden it.

The menus on pages 203 to 212 give you a list of the possible meal and snack options for the rapid-weight-loss phase of the eating plan. To know what to eat, simply follow the guidelines provided on the menu. You'll find a list of everything you need to make and prepare your meal selections directly on the menu or in the subsequent recipe section.

As a weight control specialist, I have found that for most people, the best choice for breakfast during the first phase of the diet is a protein—especially a high-calcium or light choice such as the Omelet Supreme (page 203), Savory Smoked Salmon (page 203), or Fruit and Yogurt Bliss (page 204). A protein-based breakfast takes longer to digest than a breakfast without any protein and is likely to keep you satisfied for several hours. I also like a protein breakfast because it will get you out of the habit of eating too many bad carbohydrates, such as doughnuts, bagels, white bread, or low-fiber breakfast cereals early in the day. There's growing evidence that such a breakfast may impair your body's ability to keep blood-sugar levels stable as the day wears on. In other words, your hunger increases even if you have a protein for lunch or dinner.

For the most part, the breakfast choices on the 10-Day TurboCharge Diet are quick and easy to make. However, if you're running to an appointment or have an early meeting at work, you can select one of the "On the Go" choices such as the thick and creamy Sweet Shake or Cheese Melt on GG Scandinavian Bran Crispbread (page 203). If, however, you select the Atkins' Morning Start Bar, be aware that while this choice contains protein, as do all the meal

Chef's Miriam's Quick Tips for Preparing Vegetables, Seafood, and Meat without Oil or Butter

There are many fast, easy, and healthy ways to prepare vegetables, seafood, and poultry. The following are a few of Chef Miriam's favorites.

Blanching is a great way to make vegetables. It cooks them enough to take out some of the toughness, but not so much as to take away their crispness and satisfying crunch. Quickly plunge the vegetables into boiling, lightly salted water, and cook until they are brightly colored and still crisp. This way, they will have both crunch and crispness. Often, blanched vegetables are plunged into a bowl of ice water (which stops the cooking). Blanching is a great way to prepare vegetables for a crudité platter. The veggies can be stored in the refrigerator and served to company or eaten as a snack. Drizzle with a touch of seasoned rice vinegar or a good

quality balsamic vinaigrette, if you like.

Steaming is a great method for preparing vegetables and seafood. Bring about an inch of water to boil in a medium or large saucepan (depending on the size of your steamer, water shouldn't come in contact with the food). Place the food into a steamer basket. Lower the basket into the saucepan, cover, reduce the heat, and steam the food until crisp for vegetables or tender for seafood. Season your food with a splash of lemon juice or good balsamic vinegar, chopped fresh herbs, or sliced scallions.

Grilling, indoors or out, allows for a crisp exterior and tender interior. For indoor grilling, use a stove-top or ridged grill pan (nonstick would be best) and not a skillet—otherwise, it's not grilling. Prepared spice rubs go

replacement bars I recommend, people who abuse candies may find that a similar pattern emerges with the bars. If this is your history, this item is not the best choice. Instead, consider the GG 'n Egg or Ham 'n Cheese Breakfast Sandwich, both of which you can prepare in less than 5 minutes in your microwave.

In making your selections for lunch and dinner, the best choices for rapid weight loss are the seafood and green vegetable meals. You can try the Cucumber Crabmeat Salad (page 206), or Chef Miriam's Grilled Salmon Salad (page 218). If you don't care for fish, try the

well on meat, seafood, and vegetables such as mushrooms and eggplant. You can also season your food with dried herbs such as cumin, oregano, or crushed red-pepper flakes. Or, sprinkle your food with chopped fresh herbs before or after grilling. You can toss sturdy, well-flavored vegetables such as bell peppers or onion slices with balsamic or rice vinegar and some herbs (basil) before grilling.

Stir-frying is best done by coating a pan with olive oil or Pam cooking spray (don't overcoat) and heating over medium heat for a minute. Add vegetables and a sprinkle of kosher salt to get the juices flowing and perhaps even a little dried thyme or rosemary, crumbled in your fingers, for seasoning. Then cook, tossing with two spoons, adding low-fat chicken or vegetable broth, a

mixture of broth and wine (not straight wine, not straight vinegar), or water and wine a tablespoon at a time to keep the vegetables from sticking. A juicy addition would be a chopped fresh tomato or cherry tomatoes. Season with chopped fresh herbs before serving. Very dense vegetables, such as broccoli, carrots, and cauliflower should be blanched first or sliced thinly; otherwise, they could scorch before they cook.

Poached vegetables are simmered in a layer of liquid (enough to coat the pan) until cooked. Use chicken broth and water or a mixture of broth and wine, wine and water, or mild vinegar and water. While the poaching liquid is simmering, add some smashed garlic cloves, sliced onion, strips of citrus peel, cracked black pepper, or herb sprigs for flavor before adding your food.

Ham 'n Cheese Breakfast Sandwich (page 204), Chef Miriam's Many Vegetable Omelet (page 205), or my recipe for Cold Cut Rolls (page 208).

When you peruse the lunch and dinner choices, you may notice that I often recommend bran crackers, especially the GG Scandinavian Bran Crispbread, in lieu of bread. There are many reasons for this. Bran crackers serve the same purpose as bread, give crunch without the calories, offer more nutrition for far fewer calories, provide more fiber and volume than whole grain bread, and for people who have a history of abusing bread products, they avoid the association of bread with meals. You may even discover, as have many of my clients, that you do not want to return to

How to Avoid 7 Common Kitchen Pitfalls

In many homes, kitchens are more than just a place to eat and prepare food. They're focal points, refuges—places where people meet to discuss their day, socialize, work, watch television, or chat on the telephone. Even the refrigerator has become a shrine of sorts, adorned with magnets, photos, report cards, schedules, favorite aphorisms, and reminders about important dates and events.

With so much time spent in the kitchen and its importance in the lives of so many people, the opportunities to overeat are virtually endless. So to avoid problems in the kitchen, follow these seven strategies.

1. **Avoid cooking when you're hungry.** You might end up sampling so much of what you're making that in no time at all, you'll find you've eaten several hundred calories worth of food—before you ever sit down to dinner! If you're concerned, have your 80- to 100-calorie snack before you start cooking or a low-calorie drink such as Jeff's Diet Chocolate Soda.

2. **Don't talk on the telephone or do work in the kitchen.** Doing these things encourages food grazing and mindless eating. Try to limit your "kitchen conversation" to discussions around the dining room table. If you have to work, find some place other than your kitchen to do it.

3. **Turn on the lights.** If you come into the kitchen at night, turn on as many lights as you can find (one

bread products on either the second or third parts of the diet. However, if you find that you still want bread in this phase of the eating plan, one piece of light or wheat bread (45 calories or less a slice) once or twice a week is allowed. Truth be told, my goal in this phase of the diet is really to wean you off bread since the overconsumption of bread and bread products is one of the biggest reasons why people fail on diets. I often joke with my clients that if not for the baker's oven, their great figures wouldn't have gone up in smoke!

If you decide to eat out, don't order any of the items that appear on the menu unless you know exactly how they're prepared. For example, restaurant versions of turkey, tuna, or chicken salad

recent study found that people tend to eat more in dimly lit rooms).

4. **Don't go into the kitchen when you're upset.** People sometimes eat when they're anxious, nervous, or distressed.

5. **Avoid eating while reading and watching TV.** Pleasurable activities such as reading and watching television can cause you to lose track of the amounts you're eating since your mind is often absorbed in what you're doing. Even worse, you may find yourself eating until your program is over, or you've finished reading. Sitting next to the food makes it too easy to eat extra and keeps food before your eyes all the time.

6. **Don't become the "garbage compactor."** It's not your job to finish everyone's leftovers. If you're in the habit of picking or nibbling at what remains on other people's plates, have a piece of gum, hard candy, or a Listerine Breath Strip, all of which can help keep you away from the scraps. Always keep the Listerine Breath Strips or a Halls Sugar-Free cough drop on your kitchen counter.

7. **Beware of the kitchen counter.** *Don't forget that in your house, the single most dangerous spot in terms of food control is the kitchen counter.* I've found that people invariably pick or nibble on anything that's lying on the counter—even if they're not hungry. A good rule of thumb is to keep your counter free of temptation, especially in the form of nibble or finger foods.

may contain gobs of high-fat mayonnaise or high-calorie dressing. The word "salad" in the title of a menu item is no guarantee that it'll be low in calories. Once again, ask yourself (or your server) what the salad comes with and how it is prepared.

If you find a food that comes in either water or oil, such as tuna or certain canned vegetables, always select the one that comes in water. As a general rule, oil should be limited to cooking sprays during this phase of ABC Eating. If you must have oil with your meal, limit it to 1 or 2 teaspoons of olive or canola oil on a salad or one of the recommended vegetables, *and do not use it as part of your overall food preparation*. Many of my clients who like oil find that 1 or 2 teaspoons of truffle oil goes a lot further than other oils they've tried.

Although I don't insist, it's best to avoid alcohol completely during the 10-day diet, unless it's for a special event. In that case, most of my clients find that the best choice is a small (3-ounce) glass of dry red or white wine, scotch and club soda, or vodka and club soda. Don't replace the club soda with tonic water. It's not calorie-free and could have as many calories as the alcohol. Also, don't drink on an empty stomach—and order a second, nonalcoholic drink, and alternate drinking that with the alcoholic drink.

How about fruit? The sweet taste of most fruits comes from the sugar in the fruit. Fruit sugar will not raise your blood sugar as much as table sugar and the fiber in the skin of fruits such as apples and pears may help slow down absorption (the fiber delays your stomach's ability to get to the sugar). Since I want you to get the benefits of fruit (fiber, vitamins, minerals), I've included a limited number in the 10-Day TurboCharge Diet that don't have a lot of calories and won't cause too many problems with your blood sugar, such as grapefruit, cantaloupe, apples, and strawberries. If you're a sugar-sensitive person, it's best to have it as part of a meal or as a snack that includes protein. Some of my clients who fall into the sugar-sensitive category will take half the recommended amount of fruit and combine it with a low-fat protein such as a wedge of Laughing Cow Light cheese. And be sure to eat the protein first to help control your blood sugar.

It's also a good idea to avoid fruit juices, which are frequently loaded with sugar, provide little or no fiber (except for fresh-squeezed orange juice), and can raise your blood sugar as much as a can of soda or candy bar. The only exception to this rule would be tomato juice or V8 Vegetable Juice, because I've found they act as appetite suppressants.

It's a very rare occurrence, but sometimes a client will get bored with this phase of the eating plan. If this happens to you, try shifting for several days to the B-list foods, and then go back to the 10-day diet. However, in the first 10 days, I don't recommend that you mix and match the choices in the B-list and A-list phases because it makes you lose structure. I don't want your very adaptable taste buds becoming accustomed to the higher-calorie choices offered in the second stage of the diet until you feel comfortable with your weight loss and in control of your eating. In addition, too much variety is not helpful for most people when first starting a diet.

While this phase of the eating plan is geared for 10 days, often my clients will ask when's the best time to move on to the second stage of ABC Eating. My answer is twofold. You can move to the second phase once you've lost 5 to 10 pounds. Or, you can delay shifting if you lose weight slowly or have lost weight slowly in the past. Others may elect to stay on the first phase because they feel comfortable with the structure of A-list eating or don't want the increased variety and somewhat more caloric foods of the B-list.

For health purposes, it's not recommended that you lose more than 2 pounds a week after the first 14 days. Since the 10-Day TurboCharge Diet is such a powerful plan for weight loss, some people will still be losing more than 2 pounds after the first 2 weeks. If this applies to you, it's best to add an extra fruit, a few more servings of GG & Cheese, or eat more chicken in lieu of the fruit to slow down the loss.

Always have a complete physical before going on this diet, and check with your doctor monthly while losing weight.

The 10-Day TurboCharge Diet

The core of my 10-Day TurboCharge Diet is eggs, fish, and high-calcium dairy foods such as yogurt and low-fat cheese, along with my recommended high-fiber crispbread. Many other selections are given for those who prefer other types of meals or who may need a little more variety. I cannot emphasize enough, however, that for the optimal benefit, the core foods should be selected. For each meal, an asterisk (★) will be placed against the selections that will produce the accelerated weight loss. Whatever meal you do select, you should experience significant weight loss with the 10-Day TurboCharge Diet. Enjoy!

Note on suggested serving size: When two amounts are indicated, the lower amount applies to women and the higher amount to men.

Note on high-fiber crackers: My first choice is the GG Scandinavian Bran Crispbread, since it is the only thick cracker with a mere 16 calories, 3 grams of appetite-quenching fiber, and 3 grams of carbohydrates (0 net carbs!) If you are waiting for a shipment to arrive at your local health food store or from the sources indicated in our reference section, you may *temporarily* substitute the Bran-a-Crisp, WASA Light Rye, FiberRich, or any other thick high-fiber cracker that has no more than 25 calories and at least 2 grams of fiber. All of these crackers have more calories and carbohydrates and less fiber, so I strongly recommend you only use the GGs.

Note on light cheese: My top choice of a light cheese is Laughing Cow Light, since it comes premeasured in individually wrapped triangles (each of which is only 35 calories). If you can't find Laughing Cow Light, temporarily use the Laughing Cow, because they are only 15 more calories, until you obtain the light ones from the source indicated in our reference section, or use 2 tablespoons of Alouette Cheese Spread for each Laughing Cow Light or 1 Mini Bonbel Light or Swiss Knight Light. But I strongly recommend Laughing Cow Light because it is the lowest in calories and it is instantly spreadable. Remember: Laughing Cow is wrapped and can travel with you anywhere.

Breakfast Menu

Quick and Easy Breakfast

These items may be enjoyed every day and take less than 15 minutes to prepare.

✳ Omelet Supreme

Prepare with either 4 egg whites, 1 yolk and 3 egg whites, or 6 ounces of egg substitute (e.g., Egg Beaters), and 1 slice of fat-free cheese (such as Borden's or Kraft). You may also substitute 1 tablespoon of Parmesan cheese for the fat-free cheese. If you like, you may have 1 or 2 GG Scandinavian Bran Crispbread or comparable high-fiber crackers with your meal. Prepare with Pam or olive oil cooking spray.

✳ Ham 'n Eggs

Prepare in the same way as the Omelet Supreme, and add 1 slice of light ham (Hillshire Farms or any 10- to 15-calorie light ham such as Healthy Choice) in lieu of cheese.

Cheese Melt on GG Crispbread

Melt 2 or 3 slices of fat-free cheese or 1 or 2 pieces of low-fat cheese (1 or 2 Laughing Cow Light wedges) on 2 to 4 GG Scandinavian Bran Crispbread or similar high-fiber cracker.

Apple Cottage-Cheese Delight

½ cup to 1 cup of fat-free or 1% cottage cheese on GG Scandinavian Bran Crispbread, topped with a teaspoon of apple butter or Walden Farms Apple Fruit Preserves, or a thin slice of apple, and sprinkled with cinnamon.

Gourmet Breakfast

These special choices may be enjoyed one to three times per week, especially on weekends.

Bacon 'n Eggs

Prepare with either 4 egg whites, 1 yolk and 3 egg whites, or 6 ounces of egg substitute (e.g., Better Than Eggs). Or, have 2 hard-cooked eggs. If you have scrambled eggs, add ½ cup of mushrooms and broccoli and a slice of onion. Serve with 2 slices of Butterball Thin 'n Crispy Turkey Bacon. Use a small amount of Pam or olive oil cooking spray or, better still, a coated pan without any oil.

Savory Smoked Salmon

Use 2 or 3 ounces of smoked salmon on 2 or 3 GG or other high-fiber crackers with a thick layer of fat-free cream cheese or Alouette Light Garlic & Herb or Cucumber Dill Spread. (Due to its sodium content, don't have more than 1 to 3 times a week.)

✳ *Top Choice for accelerated weight loss*

On-the-Go Breakfast

Try these delicious options when you're on the go or don't have time for a sit-down meal.

Ham 'n Cheese Breakfast Sandwich

Follow the recipe for the cheese melt but add 1 or 2 slices of light ham (Hillshire Farms or any ham that has 10 to 15 calories a slice).

Fruit and Yogurt Bliss

Take a 6- to 8-ounce cup of fat-free or light yogurt (Fage Total 2%, Dannon Lite n' Fit Carb Control, or Le Carb Yogurt) and if desired sweeten with Splenda, ½ teaspoon of cinnamon, and 1 tablespoon of sugar-free fruit preserves or 1 tablespoon of Walden Farms Preserves (0 calories). For crunch, add 1 tablespoon of Fiber One or bran cereal. You may also add 3 or 4 sliced strawberries or 3 or 4 small cubes of cantaloupe to the yogurt.

Hard-Boiled Eggs

1 or 2 hard-boiled eggs or 6 ounces of egg substitute on 2 GG crackers or similar high-fiber crackers.

Sweet Shake

One Alba shake made with fat-free milk, EAS AdvantEdge Carb Control, or Carb Solutions shake. For added flavor, you may add a few sliced strawberries and ½ teaspoon of cinnamon.

Atkins Morning Star Replacement Bar

Comes in Apple Crisp or Creamy Cinnamon, and each bar contains 160 to 170 calories.

Fast-Food Breakfast

If you decide to have breakfast away from your home, you may want to consider this low-calorie option.

McDonald's Scrambled Eggs

The scrambled eggs have 170 calories in 5.3 ounces. Do not order any sides with your eggs, especially the biscuit or bacon. You can put the eggs over my high-fiber crackers. If ordering eggs out, always emphasize no butter and no oil, just a little olive oil spray, such as Pam.

*Top Choice for accelerated weight loss

Lunch Menu

Quick and Easy Lunch

These items may be enjoyed every day.

Yogurt Jubilee

Combine a 12-ounce cup of plain, fat-free yogurt (Fage Total Yogurt) or light, low-carb yogurt with 4 table-spoons of Lipton Onion Soup mix or similar soup mix, plus dill and spices, and serve as a dip with a tray of cut-up vegetables or 2 cups of steamed green and white vegetables and/or a salad with nonfat dressing or a fla-vored balsamic vinaigrette. (For hunger control, yogurt must be com-bined with vegetables.)

Ham and Cheese Sandwich

Melt 2 or 3 slices of fat-free Amer-ican cheese or 1 or 2 triangles of Laughing Cow Light (or similar cheese such as Swiss Knight Light cheese) over 4 slices of light ham (10 to 15 calories a slice) on 4 GG or comparable high-fiber crackers. Do not use regular cheese.

Grandma's Old World Fish

Put 2 or 3 pieces of gefilte fish (in liquid) on a salad (you may add horseradish if you like). If you don't care for gefilte fish, substitute 2 to 4 ounces of smoked salmon in a tossed salad with capers.

Good Ol' Franks

2 to 3 Hebrew National 97% Fat-Free Beef Franks or Oscar Mayer Fat Free All Beef Franks (50 calories or less per frank) on a bed of sauerkraut or spinach with 2 cups of steamed low-carb green and white vegetables and/or a salad with nonfat dressing or a flavored balsamic vinaigrette. (Try grilling the franks on the George Foreman Grill.)

Louisiana Lightning

Use 1 or 2 Gorton's Blackened Cajun Fish Fillets served on a bed of spinach or 2 cups of steamed low-carb green and white vegetables. Top with Cajun spices.

GG Sandwich with Turkey and Cheddar

Prepare this delicious sandwich with 2 or 3 slices of light turkey breast (Hillshire Farms or Oscar Mayer Light), a slice of fat-free cheddar cheese (Alpine Lace), and 4 GG crackers. Add a thin layer of spicy mustard or Kraft Fat-Free Mayon-naise. Enjoy with 2 cups of steamed low-carb green and white vegetables.

Many Vegetable Omelet

Made with 4 egg whites, or 1 yolk and 3 egg whites, or 6 ounces of egg sub-stitute (e.g., Egg Beaters), and 1 slice of fat-free cheese (such as Borden's or

Kraft) or 1 ounce of fat-free feta cheese (such as President's), or 1 slice of light cheese (such as Laughing Cow Light), or 1 tablespoon of Parmesan cheese. If you like, you may have 1 or 2 bran crackers with your meal. Prepare with Pam or olive oil cooking spray or use a coated pan without oil. Enjoy with 2 cups of steamed, low-carb green and white vegetables.

GGs with Cheese and Fruit
See recipe, page 253.

Cucumber Crabmeat or Shrimp Salad
Prepare 5 or 6 ounces of crabmeat or sliced, cooked shrimp, and mix with 1 or 2 tablespoons of Kraft Fat-Free Mayonnaise, or 1 tablespoon of Hellman's Light Mayonnaise. Add chopped celery, a little chopped onion, tomato, and garlic powder, and serve on slivers of cucumbers or over a mixed green salad.

Apple Cottage-Cheese Delight
Feel free to enjoy this breakfast choice for lunch (just add 25% more cottage cheese) on 4 GGs or other bran crackers, and top with ½ to 1 teaspoon cinnamon.

Grilled Fish Salad
Those eating out may have grilled fish or shrimp with a salad or steamed vegetables. Make sure the fish is grilled dry, with no added butter or oil. See recipe, page 218.

Dilled Egg Salad
See recipe, page 221.

Gourmet Lunch

These special choices are to be used 1 or 2 times per week, especially on weekends.

Farmland Turkey or Chicken Salad
Prepare 2 to 4 ounces of white meat chicken or turkey over a tossed salad. You may add 1 tablespoon of vinaigrette, 1 tablespoon of grated Parmesan cheese, or 1 or 2 slices of Laughing Cow Light, 4 Spanish olives, 3 or 4 slivers of sun-dried tomato (packed in water), and Mrs. Dash or Cajun seasonings.

General G's Chinese Seafood
For best results, sauté or steam 4 to 6 ounces of seafood, such as shrimp, scallops, or lobster, in rice wine or broth with scallions, ginger, and garlic. *The seafood should not be sautéed in oil!* Serve with steamed Chinese vegetables prepared in the same way. For added flavor, try a little light soy or mustard sauce, or serve in a bowl with wonton soup (minus the wonton noodles). The same recipe may be prepared with white meat chicken, but it's not a first choice for accelerated weight loss.

Top Choice for accelerated weight loss

Dr. G.'s Light Pizza

Spray a cookie sheet with Pam or olive oil cooking spray. Top 3 or 4 GG crackers with 1 ounce of Calabro fat-free or Polly-O fat-free shredded mozzarella cheese, fat-free tomato sauce or paste, Ragu Pizza Sauce, mushrooms, garlic, and oregano or pizza spices. Bake until cheese melts.

Totally Tofu

Prepare the Chinese-themed dish (General G's Chinese) with 2 to 4 ounces of tofu and 1 or 2 cups of mixed steamed vegetables.

Mustard-Crumbed Chicken

See recipe, page 261.

Portobello Sandwich

Prepare 1 or 2 of the recommended veggie burgers, such as Boca or Dr. Praeger's, on slivers of portobello mushrooms topped with alfalfa sprouts. For added zest, try a little Walden Farms Fat-Free BBQ Sauce. Enjoy with a salad and/or 2 cups of steamed, low-carb, green and white vegetables.

Hearty Seafood Broth

1 to 1½ pounds of mussels or steamers made in wine and broth with mushrooms and garlic (no oil, butter, or tomato sauce).

Many Vegetable Soup

See recipe, page 216.

Pink Tuscan Tuna

Make this delicious salad with 4 to 6 ounces of water-packed chunk light tuna (which is low in mercury). Mix in a food processor with 2 tablespoons of Kraft Fat-Free Mayonnaise or 1 tablespoon of Hellman's Light Mayonnaise with 1 red pimiento pepper (water-packed only). After it's mixed, sprinkle on 1 teaspoon of crushed garlic or chopped onion and 2 tablespoons chopped tomato. Place over a tossed salad or uncooked spinach, and top with chives, 1 tablespoon of grated Parmesan cheese, and 1 tablespoon of cut-up sun-dried tomato (not packed in oil).

Leaning Vegetable Stacks

See recipe, page 220.

Better Than Deli Tuna Salad

See recipe, page 217.

On-the-Go Lunch

Try these delicious choices when you're on the go or don't have time for a sit-down meal.

Pria Bar (approximately 170 calories)

GG Veggie-Cheese Crunch

Takes only 4 minutes to prepare. See recipe, page 253.

2 Sweet Shakes

Double the breakfast amount.
Note: Many other chain restaurants offer garden salads with chicken or

seafood. This is an option as long as you choose one in the 200- to 225-calorie range and use their fat-free dressing.

Fast-Food Lunch

Heavenly Roll

8 to 10 pieces of sashimi or cucumber sashimi (fish rolled in cucumber skin). Serve with wasabi mustard and a light soy sauce. Add a bowl of miso soup (it's high in sodium, so don't weigh yourself for 24 hours).

Cold-Cut Rolls

Start with large lettuce leaves. Place 8 to 10 slices of light cold cuts (Oscar Mayer Light, Hillshire Farms, or Healthy Choice) on the leaves, and roll around pickle spears, cucumber, or zucchini sticks.

McDonald's Chicken Caesar Salad

Replace the Caesar dressing with ½ pack of their Newman's Balsamic Vinaigrette.

Subway Mediterranean Chicken Salad

Only with their Kraft Fat-Free Italian Dressing

Burger King Fire-Grilled Shrimp Salad

Fire-Grilled Chicken Garden Salad

Only with their Hidden Valley Fat-Free Ranch Dressing

Arby's Asian Sesame Chicken Salad

Without almonds, noodles, sesame dressing, and only with their fat-free Italian dressing

✳Top Choice for accelerated weight loss

Dinner Menu

Quick and Easy Dinner

These items may be enjoyed every day. If you prefer, any lunch entrée may be enjoyed in lieu of dinner.

Frozen Low-Carb Dinners

Select any frozen entrée (such as Stouffers, Weight Watchers, or Healthy Choice) that's low-carb and contains no more than 300 calories. Pick the new low carb entrées where rice, potatoes, and pastas have been replaced with lower-carb vegetables. Have a big salad and additional cups of steamed low-carb, green and white vegetables.

Dr. G's Chicken Parmesan

Start with 1 or 2 low-fat, Italian-style breaded chicken cutlets that are pre-cooked (Perdue Low-Fat Breaded Italian Cutlets or Tyson Italian-Style Tasty Selections Boneless and Skinless Chicken Breast). Spray a baking sheet (pan) with Pam or olive oil cooking spray. Top the cutlet(s) with fat-free tomato sauce or Ragu Pizza Sauce, and 1 ounce of Polly-O fat-free or Calabro fat-free shredded mozzarella cheese, garlic powder or crushed garlic, and a little parsley. Preheat your oven to 350°F, and heat briefly until the cheese melts. Serve with 2 cups of steamed vegetables and a salad with nonfat dressing or flavored balsamic vinaigrette. If you wish to prepare your own, use 4 to 6 ounces of chicken breast.

Grilled Fish or Seafood

Prepare with 4 to 6 ounces of white meat fish or seafood such as shrimp, lobster, or crabmeat. Serve with 2 cups of steamed vegetables and a tossed salad.

Scallop and Vegetable Packets

See recipe, page 236.

Dr. G.'s World Famous Zucchini/Eggplant Parmigiana

See recipe, page 222. Women may eat ½ to ⅔ of the recipe. Men can eat ⅔ or the entire recipe (it's high in sodium).

America's Most Delicious Veggie Burgers

Prepare two Dr. Praeger's Veggie Burgers or Boca Burgers, and serve on a bed of spinach with a cup of steamed vegetables or a bowl of my recommended soups. (Use burgers that are 80 to 100 calories each.) For added flavor, try a tablespoon of Walden Farms Calorie-Free Barbecue Sauce.

Good Ol' Franks

Increase the lunch menu to 3 or 4 franks.

Dr. G's Chef's Salad Light
Make with 3 to 5 ounces of sliced fresh turkey, 1 slice of light Swiss cheese, such as Alpine Lace (not more than 80 calories a slice), and 1 or 2 slices of my recommended light ham. For a dressing, try balsamic vinegar mixed with lemon and mustard. Have with 2 cups of low-carb green and white vegetables.

Dr. G's Stracchiatella Soup
See recipe, page 213.

Gourmet Dinner

These items may be enjoyed every day.

Creole Crumbed Shrimp
See recipe, page 225.

Sticks of Fish
Prepare simply with 4 or 5 Van de Kamp's Crisp or Healthy Choice Original Breaded Fish Sticks or comparable brand, frozen fish sticks. Serve with 2 cups of steamed asparagus and 1 tablespoon of low-cal dressing.

Fish n' Chips
Made with Sticks of Fish (see above) and Oven "Fried" Zucchini chips (see recipe, page 219)

Dr. G's Shrimp Scampi
Start by sautéing 6 to 8 ounces of shrimp in a pan sprayed with 1 or 2 sprays of Pam or Weight Watchers

Butter Spray with a little fat-free chicken broth. Add 2 or 3 tablespoons of crushed garlic with a little wine and a sprinkle of parsley for added flavor. Follow up with five sprays of I Can't Believe It's Not Butter spray.

Mussels with Soy and Sherry
See recipe, page 235.

Roasted Sage-Lemon Salmon
See recipe, page 233.

Seafood in Brodo
See recipe, page 232.

Chef Miriam's Dinners

Grilled Spice-Rubbed Pork Tenderloin with Cucumber-Yogurt Sauce
See recipe, page 258.

Yucatan-Styled Grilled Swordfish
Note: Swordfish is high in mercury and should not be consumed more than 1 or 2 times a week maximum, and not at all by pregnant or nursing women.
See recipe, page 238.

Oven-Steamed Salmon Hong Kong–Style
See recipe, page 230.

Seafood Salad Positano
See recipe, page 234.

Solar Harvest Dinners

Solar Harvest's Roasted Organic Turkey Breast
See recipe, page 286.

Top Choice for accelerated weight loss

Snacks and Minimeals

Women should have a maximum of two snacks or minimeals per day. Men may have up to three. One of those snacks or minimeals is required in the critical late afternoon to early evening period of 3 to 5 P.M. Others may be enjoyed in the midmorning, evening, or right before dinner to prevent any hunger. Or you may elect to omit the additional snack(s) and use your "free foods" instead. The critical determinant is that you should avoid being hungry at any time during the day.

Where two amounts are indicated, women should have the lower amount and men the larger amount.

Yogurt: Fage Total Yogurt 0% or comparable fat-free yogurt (Dannon Carb Control, Le Carb Yogurt)

Total Yogurt is 80 calories; adjust the other yogurt to get between 80 and 100 calories per serving.

Alba Fit 'n Frosty Shake

Prepare with water, Jeff's Diet Chocolate or Vanilla Soda, or coffee. This is my first choice for a snack.

Spicy Hot V-8 Juice or a low-sodium vegetable or tomato juice 6-ounce serving

Grapefruit

3 halves = 1 snack. If you select this snack, you should have half a grapefruit with each meal. Since this is a snack designed to be a calorie-budget stretcher, it works best in that capacity immediately after a meal. Women should avoid a large grapefruit. (Do not have more than 3 halves of grapefruit per day.)

Bowl of Soup

A serving of Health Valley Fat-Free Soups, Tabatchnick's Frozen Soups, or the portable envelope of Lipton's Cup-a-Soup have 70 to 80 calories and may be enjoyed with 1 high-fiber cracker (not more than 25 calories).

Cheese Omelet

2 egg whites and 1 slice of 30-calorie fat-free cheese or 1 tablespoon of Parmesan cheese mixed with cut-up low-carb, green and white vegetables. You may omit the cheese.

Dr. G's Light Pizza

See recipe, page 207. Women may have 2 cracker pizzas and men may have up to 3.

Hot Dogs

1 or 2 light hot dogs (Hebrew National 97% Fat-Free Hot Dogs, Oscar Mayer Fat-Free All-Beef Hot Dogs, or a comparable 50-calorie light hot dog) on a bed of sauerkraut or 1 cup of steamed low carb green and white vegetables.

Dr. G's BLT

2 GG Scandinavian Bran Crispbread or comparable high-fiber crackers, lettuce, a thin slice of tomato, 2 slices of Butterball Thin 'N Crispy Turkey Bacon, and a thin spread of Kraft Fat-Free Mayonnaise.

2 Laughing Cow Cheese Wedges or 1 Polly-O Part-Skim Mozzarella Stick

Yogurt Crunch 'n Berry

6 ounces of Total 0% Yogurt or comparable low-carb (80 calories or less per serving) yogurt sprinkled with 2 teaspoons of Fiber One cereal, one sliced medium-size strawberry, and Splenda.

Chocolate Pudding

6 ounces of Total 0% Yogurt or a comparable low-carb, 80-calories-per-serving yogurt. Mix with 2 or 3 tablespoons of Walden Farms No-Calorie Chocolate Syrup or Chocolate Dip or No-Carb Gourmet Chocolate Syrup.

Cappuccino with Fat-Free Milk (8-ounce serving)

If you would like a sweet accompaniment, try one of the high-fiber crackers and a tablespoon of Walden Farms Calorie-Free Fruit Preserves.

Fat-Free Cottage Cheese (4 to 6 ounces)

You can mix cottage cheese and 1 tablespoon of Walden Farms Calorie-Free Fruit Preserves.

Crackers 'n Cold Cuts Sandwich

2 GG Scandinavian Bran Crispbreads or comparable high-fiber cracker such as WASA Light Rye or Fiber-Rich with 2 or 3 slices of any light cold cut (10 to 15 calories per slice) topped with mustard or a thin spread of Kraft No-Fat Mayonnaise. (Optional: lettuce and a thin slice of tomato).

Shrimp or Crabmeat Cocktail

4 to 6 medium-size shrimp or 4 or 5 ounces of crabmeat topped with Walden's No-Calorie Seafood Sauce.

One Hard-Boiled Egg

You can chop the egg over a green salad, or you can use 4 ounces of egg substitute (preferably with cut-up vegetables or salad).

Micro-Spice Butternut Squash

See recipe, page 241.

---

*Top Choice for accelerated weight loss

Free Foods

The following foods are unlimited unless otherwise indicated:

- Coffee
- Tea
- Tomato juice (4 ounces; 1 to 2 times per day; preferably low salt)
- Diet soda
- All condiments
- Green and white low-calorie, low-carb vegetables. This does not include peas, onions, the squash family, potatoes, jicama, avocado, and obviously tomatoes, carrots, beans, chick peas, peas, and lentils.

The following foods are free if used as indicated, with the lower amount for women and the higher amount for men:

- 2 egg whites per day (may be combined with free green and white vegetables to make an omelet or vegetable soufflé)
- ½ grapefruit a day (eaten with your heaviest caloric meal of the day)
- 2 GG crackers or one of the substitute crackers such as Bran-a-Crisp or WASA Light Rye
- 1 or 2 fruit ice pops such as Lifesaver Popsicles that are 10 to 18 calories; not juice pops
- Diet Sugar-Free Jell-O or Gelatin
- Walden Farms Calorie-Free Chocolate Syrup and Chocolate Dip
- 1 sugar-free gum (e.g., Sugar Busters, Dentyne Fire). Have no more than 3 or 4 pieces per day.
- Yoplait, Weight Watchers, or Tofutti chocolate mousse pops that are a maximum of 30 to 40 calories may be enjoyed at night, not as an afternoon snack
- 1 cup of fat-free, low-salt chicken broth (may be combined with the green and white vegetables such as spinach or cabbage to make a free vegetable soup). You can even add one of your free egg whites to the boiling soup to make an instant egg-drop soup, or add cooked, drained spinach to have an Italian spinach soup (Stracchiatella).

You can enjoy a maximum of two or three of the following as needed:

- Jeff's Diet Chocolate or Vanilla Soda (20 calories)
- Swiss Miss Diet Hot Chocolate (10 calories each)
- Carnation Diet Hot Chocolate (Do not buy any hot chocolate with more than 25 calories.)

Keep in mind that the FDA allows foods that are less than 5 calories per serving to be classified as having zero calories.

Amazing Lemony Soup
with Crab and Vegetables

Prep: 5 minutes • Cook: 9 minutes

This soup is amazing because it's so easy, so delicious, and so low in calories. Cooked shredded chicken could be used instead of the crab.

1 can (14.5 ounces) fat-free reduced-sodium chicken broth

1 garlic clove, peeled and cut in half

1 cup sliced mushrooms (use presliced)

½ cup thinly sliced zucchini

1½ packed cups baby spinach

½ cup (2 ounces) lump crabmeat, picked over

¼ teaspoon grated lemon zest

1 tablespoon fresh lemon juice

In a medium saucepan, combine the broth and garlic. Cover and bring to a boil over high heat. Add the mushrooms and zucchini; reduce the heat to medium, cover, and simmer until the vegetables are tender, about 3 minutes.

Stir in the spinach and cook just until wilted, about 30 seconds. Remove from the heat and stir in the crab, lemon zest, and juice. Discard the garlic. Serve immediately.

Makes 1 serving (2¼ cups)

Per serving: 140 calories, 1.5 g fat, 0 g saturated fat, 19 g protein, 14 g carbohydrates, 5 g dietary fiber, 45 mg cholesterol, 890 mg sodium

Dilled Cucumber and Yogurt Soup

Prep: 10 minutes

This soup is very refreshing on a warm day—best yet, no cooking is necessary. Sip from a mug and accompany with a GG Scandinavian Bran Crispbread.

1 cup sliced hothouse cucumber

2 tablespoons chopped sweet onion

1 tablespoon snipped fresh dill

1 teaspoon rice wine vinegar

$\frac{1}{2}$ small garlic clove

$\frac{1}{4}$ teaspoon dried mint, crumbled

$\frac{1}{8}$ teaspoon salt

$\frac{3}{4}$ cup plain nonfat yogurt

Freshly ground black pepper, to taste

Put the cucumber, onion, dill, vinegar, garlic, mint, and salt in a food processor and process until very finely chopped.

Add the yogurt and process until smooth. Season to taste with pepper. Serve immediately, with a slice of cucumber floating on top, or cover and chill until ready to serve.

Makes 1 serving (1$\frac{1}{2}$ cups)

Per serving: 100 calories, 0 g fat, 0 g saturated fat, 9 g protein, 20 g carbohydrates, 1 g dietary fiber, 5 mg cholesterol, 400 mg sodium

Many Vegetable Soup

Prep: 15 minutes ● Cook: 23 minutes

You'll want to keep this soup on hand for lunches and snacks. If you like, add a little protein to each bowl with some chopped hard-cooked egg white or a tablespoon of grated Parmesan or shredded mozzarella.

> 3 cans (14.5 ounces each) fat-free reduced-sodium chicken broth
> 1 cup thinly sliced celery, with some leaves
> 1 small onion, halved and thinly sliced
> 1 garlic clove, minced
> 2 teaspoons chopped fresh thyme leaves
> 2 cups thinly sliced cauliflower florets
> 1 cup cut green beans, $\frac{1}{2}$-inch pieces
> 2 cups diagonally sliced asparagus
> 2 cups thinly sliced yellow summer squash or zucchini
> $\frac{1}{4}$ teaspoon salt

In a Dutch oven or large saucepan, combine the broth, celery, onion, garlic, and thyme. Cover and bring to a boil over high heat.

Stir in the cauliflower and green beans. Reduce the heat to medium, cover, and simmer until crisp-tender, 5 minutes. Stir in the asparagus, squash, and salt. Cover and simmer until the vegetables are tender, about 5 minutes longer. Serve hot.

Makes 4 servings (8 cups)

Per serving: 80 calories, 0.5 g fat, 0 g saturated fat, 7 g protein, 13 g carbohydrates, 4 g dietary fiber, 0 mg cholesterol, 670 mg sodium

Better Than Deli Tuna Salad

Prep: 10 minutes

Fresher, leaner, and full of crunch—you'll swear off deli tuna salad after
enjoying this slimmed-down version. Serve on a bed of crisp mixed greens
spritzed with lemon juice or balsamic vinegar, or spread the salad on GG
Scandinavian Bran Crispbreads.

1 can (3 ounces) water-packed tuna, drained and flaked

1 hard-cooked egg white, chopped

¼ cup each finely chopped red and green bell peppers

¼ cup chopped celery

2 to 3 tablespoons chopped dill pickle

1½ tablespoons light mayonnaise

1 tablespoon chopped red onion

Salt and freshly ground pepper to taste

In a salad bowl, combine all ingredients and stir with a fork to blend
well. Serve immediately, or cover and refrigerate until ready to serve.

Makes 1 serving (1½ cups)

*Per serving: 230 calories, 10 g fat, 2 g saturated fat, 25 g protein,
9 g carbohydrates, 1 g dietary fiber, 45 mg cholesterol, 810 mg sodium*

Grilled Salmon Salad

Prep: 6 minutes • Cook: 14 minutes • Cooling time: 10 minutes

Fresh is best but a 3.75-ounce can of salmon can be used in a pinch. Don't discard the tiny soft bones from the canned salmon; they're full of calcium. Serve this salad on a bed of mixed greens, with vegetable sticks or GG Scandinavian Bran Crispbreads. (*Note:* You can substitute another type of fish for the salmon if you desire.)

One 3- to 4-ounce skinned salmon fillet
1/8 teaspoon coarsely ground black pepper
Pinch salt
1 hard-cooked egg white, chopped
1/3 cup chopped cucumber
1/4 cup chopped yellow, orange, or red bell pepper
1 scallion, thinly sliced
1 tablespoon coarsely chopped pimiento-stuffed green olives
1 tablespoon fat-free mayonnaise
1 teaspoon grainy mustard

Coat a stovetop grill pan or a small nonstick skillet with olive oil cooking spray. Heat over medium heat for 2 minutes.

Season the salmon with pepper and salt. Place on the grill pan or in the skillet and cook until lightly browned on the outside and just opaque in the thickest part, 2 to 4 minutes per side. Transfer to a plate and let stand 10 minutes to cool.

Break the salmon into coarse flakes. Put in a salad bowl and mix in the egg white, cucumber, bell pepper, scallion, olives, mayonnaise, and mustard. Serve immediately, or cover and refrigerate until ready to serve.

Makes 1 serving

Per serving: 270 calories, 14 g fat, 2.5 g saturated fat, 27 g protein, 8 g carbohydrates, 2 g dietary fiber, 70 mg cholesterol, 690 mg sodium

Oven "Fried" Zucchini

Prep: 5 minutes • Cook: 20 minutes

There are two ways to do this: You can sliver the zucchini in a food processor fitted with the slicing blade, and you'll get very thin "chips." Some will bake up crisp; some will be meltingly soft. Or you can make thin wedges, which will be a touch crispy on the outside and tender on the inside. Both are good. And both need to be eaten hot from the oven. Sprinkle a touch of Cajun seasoning over the zucchini when it comes out of the oven, if you like.

> 2 medium zucchini (about 1 pound), trimmed and cut into
> wedges ¼ inch wide and 4 inches long, or halved lengthwise
> (to fit in the food processor's feed tube)
> 3 large egg whites
> ¼ teaspoon salt

Preheat the oven to 500°F. If making wedges, coat a large heavy baking sheet with olive oil cooking spray; if making slivers, you'll need to prepare 2 baking sheets.

In a large bowl, whisk the egg whites and salt until frothy. Add the zucchini and toss to coat well; let stand for 5 minutes.

Arrange the zucchini wedges in single layers with a cut side down on the prepared baking sheet, letting the excess egg white drip into the bowl. Arrange the slivers in single layers on the 2 sheets, without worrying if some overlap. Mist the zucchini with olive oil cooking spray.

Bake the wedges, turning once to the other cut side, until golden, about 15 minutes. Bake the slivers without turning, moving the pans to the opposite racks halfway though baking, until lightly browned in spots, about 12 minutes.

Let zucchini stand on the baking sheet(s) for a minute after removing from the oven. Scrape onto a plate and serve hot.

Makes 2 servings

Per serving: 60 calories, 0 g fat, 0 g saturated fat, 8 g protein, 8 g carbohydrates, 2 g dietary fiber, 0 mg cholesterol, 400 mg sodium

Leaning Vegetable Stacks

Prep: 15 minutes • Cook: 37 minutes

Your diet-conscious friends and family will love this satisfying dish. These stacks lean slightly, not unlike the Tower of Pisa.

3 large garlic cloves, minced

2 tablespoons chopped fresh rosemary

1 tablespoon chopped fresh oregano

$\frac{1}{2}$ teaspoon freshly ground black pepper

$\frac{1}{4}$ teaspoon salt

4 medium portabello mushroom caps (4 inches), wiped clean, stems cut out

Four $\frac{1}{2}$-inch slices peeled eggplant, cut crosswise

1 large red bell pepper, cut in thin strips

2 medium tomatoes, each cored and cut in 4 slices

$\frac{3}{4}$ cup nonfat ricotta cheese

1 cup shredded part-skim mozzarella cheese

Preheat the broiler. Coat 2 rimmed baking sheets with olive oil cooking spray.

In a cup, mix the garlic, rosemary, oregano, pepper, and salt.

On one of the baking sheets, place the mushrooms and eggplant. Mist with olive oil cooking spray and sprinkle with some of the herb mixture. Turn the vegetables over and repeat.

Place the bell pepper strips in a small bowl and toss with some herb mixture. Arrange the tomatoes on the other prepared baking sheet; sprinkle the remaining herb mixture on both sides.

Broil the mushrooms and eggplant 3 to 5 inches from the heat until lightly browned, about 5 minutes. Turn and broil 5 minutes longer, until the eggplant is tender (mushrooms won't be done). Transfer the eggplant to a plate.

Place the bell pepper on the sheet next to the mushrooms. Broil, turning mushrooms and bell pepper often, until tender, 4 to 6 minutes. Remove from the heat.

Broil the tomatoes without turning, until heated through, about 5 minutes. Remove from the heat. Turn the oven to 425°F.

Prepare the stacks like this: On a baking sheet, place the mushrooms open side up. Fill each with 3 tablespoons ricotta. Arrange an eggplant slice and 2 tomato slices overlapping slightly on the mushrooms. Sprinkle with the bell pepper strips and mozzarella. Bake until hot and the cheese has melted, 4 to 6 minutes. Serve immediately.

Makes 4 servings

Per serving: 180 calories, 5 g fat, 3 g saturated fat, 14 g protein, 18 g carbohydrates, 2 g dietary fiber, 25 mg cholesterol, 340 mg sodium

Dilled Egg Salad

Prep: 12 minutes

If you don't care for dill, add parsley or a pinch of a dried herb you like. Serve with GG Scandinavian Bran Crispbreads and/or steamed broccoli. Add a fruit that's allowed and you have an entire meal.

> **1 hard-cooked egg, chopped (can use just the white), plus 3 hard-cooked egg whites, chopped**
> **¼ cup finely chopped celery**
> **2 tablespoons chopped sweet white onion**
> **2 tablespoons snipped fresh dill**
> **2 tablespoons fat-free mayonnaise**
> **1 tablespoon chopped fresh tomato**
> **½ teaspoon Dijon mustard**
> **⅛ teaspoon each salt and freshly ground black pepper**

In a salad bowl, combine all ingredients and stir with a fork to blend well. Serve immediately or cover and refrigerate until ready to serve.

Makes 1 serving (1¼ cups)

Per serving: 170 calories, 6 g fat, 2 g saturated fat, 18 g protein, 9 g carbohydrates, 1 g dietary fiber, 215 mg cholesterol, 810 mg sodium

Dr. G's World Famous Low-Calorie Zucchini/Eggplant Parmigiana

Prep: 12 minutes • Cook: 37 minutes

While dining on this festive fare, I suggest serving a crisp green salad tossed with low-fat vinaigrette. If you like, add 2 cups sliced white button or cremini mushrooms that have been sautéed in a nonstick pan with 1 tablespoon white wine. To make the meal truly memorable, play some Italian music in the background—an opera by Verdi would be most appropriate.

See the Dining for One version opposite.

> 2 teaspoons Italian dried herb seasoning
>
> ¼ teaspoon salt
>
> ¼ teaspoon crushed red pepper flakes
>
> ¼ teaspoon garlic powder
>
> 1 medium eggplant (about 1 pound), peeled and cut lengthwise into ½-inch slices
>
> 2 medium zucchini (about 1 pound), cut lengthwise into ½-inch slices
>
> 1 cup fat-free or low-fat marinara sauce
>
> 1 cup (4 ounces) shredded fat-free or part-skim mozzarella cheese
>
> ¼ cup freshly grated Parmesan cheese

Preheat the broiler. Coat a heavy baking sheet and a 13 × 9-inch glass baking dish with olive oil cooking spray.

In a cup, mix the herb seasoning, salt, red pepper flakes, and garlic powder. Arrange the eggplant slices on the prepared baking sheet; mist lightly with olive oil cooking spray and sprinkle with some herb mixture. Turn and repeat on the other side.

Broil 3 to 5 inches from the heat, turning once, until lightly browned and very tender, 8 to 10 minutes. Arrange in a single layer in the prepared baking dish.

Arrange the zucchini on the baking sheet. Spray and season as for the eggplant. Broil until tender (it won't really brown), 8 to 10 minutes. Arrange over the eggplant. Turn the oven to 450°F.

Spoon the sauce over the vegetables, spreading it evenly. Sprinkle evenly with the cheeses. Bake, uncovered, until heated and bubbly, about 10 minutes.

Makes 4 servings

Per serving: 130 calories, 2 g fat, 1 g saturated fat, 13 g protein, 16 g carbohydrates, 2 g dietary fiber, 5 mg cholesterol, 640 mg sodium

Dining for One

$\frac{1}{2}$ teaspoon Italian dried herb seasoning

Pinch salt

Pinch crushed red pepper flakes

Pinch garlic powder

2- or 3$\frac{1}{2}$-inch lengthwise slices peeled eggplant

2- or 3$\frac{1}{2}$-inch lengthwise slices zucchini

$\frac{1}{4}$ cup fat-free or low-fat marinara sauce

$\frac{1}{4}$ cup shredded fat-free or part-skim mozzarella cheese

1 tablespoon freshly grated Parmesan cheese

Preheat the broiler. Coat a heavy baking sheet and a small baking dish (about 8 × 5 inches) with olive oil cooking spray.

In a cup, mix the herbs, salt, red pepper flakes, and garlic powder. Arrange the eggplant and zucchini on the prepared baking sheet; mist lightly with olive oil cooking spray, and sprinkle with some herb mixture. Turn and repeat on the other side.

Broil 3 inches to 5 inches from the heat, turning once, until very tender, 8 to 10 minutes. Arrange in the prepared baking dish. Turn the oven to 425°F.

Top the vegetables with the sauce, spreading it evenly; sprinkle with the cheeses. Bake, uncovered, until heated and bubbly, about 10 minutes.

Green and White Dip

Prep: 2 minutes • **Cook: 6 minutes**

Serve this as a hot entrée or spread it on cucumber slices or bell pepper wedges for an appetizer.

1 cup frozen cut-leaf spinach (from a bag)
2 tablespoons water
½ cup fat-free ricotta cheese
¼ teaspoon Italian dried herb seasoning
Pinch salt
Pinch garlic powder
2 tablespoons shredded part-skim mozzarella cheese

In a small, deep, microwave-safe bowl or dish, place the spinach and water. Cover with waxed paper or vented plastic wrap. Microwave on High for 1 minute, until defrosted.

Drain in a sieve, pressing out the excess moisture. Return to the cooking dish.

With a fork, mix in the ricotta, herb seasoning, salt, and garlic powder. Spread flat in the dish.

Cover with waxed paper or vented plastic wrap and microwave on High for 1½ minutes, until heated and slightly puffed. Sprinkle with the mozzarella and microwave, uncovered, 15 to 30 seconds longer, until the cheese has melted. Let stand a few moments before serving.

Makes 1 serving (¾ cup)

Per serving: 200 calories, 3.5 g fat, 1.5 g saturated fat, 21 g protein, 21 g carbohydrates, 7 g dietary fiber, 30 mg cholesterol, 690 mg sodium

Creole Crumbed Shrimp

Prep: 10 minutes ● Cook: 33 minutes

Don't try to crush the GG Crispbreads in a food processor; it doesn't work too well. Instead, crumble them up with your hands, put them in a resealable plastic freezer bag, and crush with a rolling pin for a super aerobic workout. This goes fast if you buy the shrimp already peeled and deveined. If you like spicy, use the larger amount of seasoning and Tabasco and/or serve with additional Tabasco. As a variation, you can substitute 1½ pounds white-fish fillets for the shrimp and reduce baking time to 10 minutes.

    4 large egg whites
    3 to 4 teaspoons Creole spice blend
    2 teaspoons grated lime zest
    ½ to 1 teaspoon Tabasco sauce
    ⅛ teaspoon salt
    10 GG Scandinavian Bran Crispbreads, ground to crumbs by
        hand (see above), about 1 cup
    1½ pounds peeled and deveined large shrimp, tails left on
    Lime wedges (optional)

Preheat the oven to 400°F. Coat 2 heavy or nonstick baking sheets with olive oil cooking spray.

In a large bowl, whisk the egg whites until foamy. Beat in the Creole spice blend, lime zest, Tabasco, and salt. Place the Crispbread crumbs in a pie plate.

Place the shrimp in the egg white mixture and toss to coat. One at a time, roll a shrimp in the crumbs, pressing them lightly onto the surface so the crumbs adhere. Arrange the crumbed shrimp in single layers on the prepared baking sheets.

Mist the shrimp lightly with olive oil cooking spray. Bake until the shrimp are just opaque in the thickest part, 16 to 18 minutes.

Serve hot with lime wedges, if you like.

Makes 4 servings

Per serving: 220 calories, 2.5 g fat, 0 g saturated fat, 36 g protein, 9 g carbohydrates, 8 g dietary fiber, 225 mg cholesterol, 800 mg sodium

Baked Sole with Key West Slaw

Prep: 12 minutes • Cook: 20 minutes

Normally mild-flavored, sole gets zing from a Cajun-style mix of spices. If sole is not available, choose flounder, tilapia, orange roughy, or grouper instead—but remember that thicker fillets will take longer to cook. The slaw can be tossed together a few hours ahead, but it's best eaten the day it's prepared.

For the slaw:
>   ¼ cup fat-free mayonnaise
>   ½ teaspoon grated lime zest
>   ½ teaspoon grated orange zest
>   2 tablespoons fresh lime juice
>   ¼ teaspoon coarsely ground black pepper
>   ⅛ teaspoon salt
>   3 cups bagged tricolor slaw mix (cabbage, carrots, and red cabbage)
>   1 cup thin red or yellow bell pepper strips, each cut in half
>   2 tablespoons chopped sweet white onion

For the sole:
>   1¾ pounds sole fillets, cut in half along the center seam, bones at top removed
>   1 tablespoon fresh lime juice
>   ½ teaspoon paprika
>   ½ teaspoon salt
>   ¼ teaspoon dried thyme
>   Pinch each garlic powder and cayenne pepper

To make the slaw: In a medium bowl, whisk the mayonnaise, lime and orange zests, lime juice, pepper, and salt until blended. Add the slaw mix, bell pepper, and onion and mix with a fork. Set aside or cover and refrigerate until ready to serve.

To make the sole: Preheat the oven to 400°F. Coat a rimmed baking sheet with olive oil cooking spray.

Place the sole on the prepared baking sheet, folding the thin ends underneath, and drizzle the fillets with the lime juice. In a cup, mix the paprika, salt, thyme, garlic powder, and cayenne. Sprinkle evenly over the sole, spreading it with your fingers.

Bake the sole until it just flakes and is opaque in the thickest part, 10 to 12 minutes. Transfer the sole to plates, spooning any juices over, and serve with the slaw.

Makes 4 servings (3 cups slaw)

Per serving: 220 calories, 3 g fat, 0.5 g saturated fat, 39 g protein, 9 g carbohydrates, 1 g dietary fiber, 95 mg cholesterol, 660 mg sodium

Dr. G's Renowned Crabmeat-Stuffed Mushrooms

Prep: 8 minutes • Cook: 23 minutes

I like to serve six to eight of these delightful mushrooms as a light main dish. I also serve a few of them as a first course when entertaining friends.

> **16 large white stuffing mushrooms, stems pulled out**
> **1½ cups (6 ounces) lump crabmeat, picked over**
> **3 tablespoons chopped fresh Italian parsley**
> **3 tablespoons chopped scallions**
> **3 tablespoons grated fresh Parmesan cheese**
> **1 tablespoon vermouth or dry white wine**
> **1 garlic clove, minced**
> **⅛ teaspoon freshly ground black pepper**
> **½ cup shredded part-skim or nonfat mozzarella cheese**

Preheat the oven to 375°F. Coat a 13 x 9-inch baking pan with olive oil cooking spray. Arrange the mushrooms open side up in the prepared pan.

In a medium bowl, lightly mix together the crabmeat, parsley, scallions, Parmesan, vermouth or wine, garlic, and pepper with a fork.

Stuff the mixture into the mushrooms. Sprinkle with the mozzarella.

Bake until the mushrooms are tender and start to release juices and the cheese has melted, 15 to 18 minutes. Serve hot.

Makes 16 stuffed mushrooms (1½ cups stuffing)

Per serving: 35 calories, 1 g fat, 0.5 g saturated fat, 4 g protein, 2 g carbohydrates, 0 g dietary fiber, 15 mg cholesterol, 70 mg sodium

Broiled Snapper with Orange and Scallions

Prep: 7 minutes • Marinate: 30 minutes • Cook: 10 minutes

Serve this succulent dish with an assortment of steamed vegetables, perhaps asparagus, green beans, and yellow summer squash. Any white-fleshed fish will work here: Try bass, thick sole fillets, halibut, or tilapia. Be sure to sprinkle the scallions over the fish the moment it comes out of the broiler so they'll soften and mellow.

Four 7-ounce skinned red snapper fillets

1 teaspoon grated orange zest

2 tablespoons fresh orange juice

1 garlic clove, minced

1½ teaspoons chopped fresh rosemary

¼ teaspoon salt

⅛ teaspoon freshly ground black pepper

Pinch crushed red pepper flakes

3 tablespoons thinly sliced scallions

Arrange the snapper in a single layer in a shallow dish. In a small bowl, mix the orange zest and juice, garlic, rosemary, salt, black pepper, and red pepper flakes. Spoon the mixture evenly over both sides of the snapper, spreading it with a spoon. Cover and marinate at cool room temperature or in the refrigerator for 30 minutes.

Preheat the broiler. Coat a rimmed baking sheet with olive oil cooking spray.

Transfer the snapper to the prepared baking sheet and scrape any remaining marinade onto the fish as well.

Broil 4 to 6 inches from the heat until the fish is just opaque in the thickest part, 5 to 8 minutes. Remove from the heat and immediately sprinkle with the scallions. Serve.

Makes 4 servings

Per serving: 210 calories, 3 g fat, 0.5 g saturated fat, 41 g protein, 2 g carbohydrates, 0 g dietary fiber, 75 mg cholesterol, 270 mg sodium

Oven-Poached Halibut
with Cucumber and Celery

Prep: 13 minutes • Cook: 30 minutes

You can prepare this soothing dish with any thick, fine-textured white fish, such as cod (but not scrod), tilefish, or red snapper. The celery and thyme add richness to the poaching broth, without butter or oil. The cucumber is an unusual addition that we think you will enjoy. It's an entirely different vegetable once cooked.

$1\frac{1}{2}$ cups fat-free reduced-sodium chicken broth

$\frac{1}{4}$ cup dry vermouth or white wine

$1\frac{1}{2}$ cups thin half-moon slices peeled hothouse cucumber

1 cup thinly sliced tender celery stalks, with some leaves

1 cup thinly sliced leek, well washed

2 teaspoons coarsely chopped fresh thyme leaves

$\frac{1}{4}$ teaspoon salt

$\frac{1}{4}$ teaspoon freshly ground black pepper

$1\frac{3}{4}$ pounds skinned halibut fillet, cut in 8 equal pieces

Preheat the oven to 425°F. Set out a large, deep ovenproof skillet (wrap skillet handle with heavy-duty foil if it is not ovenproof).

In the skillet, stir together the broth, vermouth or wine, cucumber, celery, leek, 1 teaspoon thyme, and ⅛ teaspoon each salt and pepper. Bring to a boil over high heat. Reduce the heat to medium-low, cover, and simmer until the vegetables are tender, about 10 minutes.

Meanwhile, season the halibut with the remaining 1 teaspoon thyme and remaining ⅛ teaspoon each salt and pepper.

Arrange the halibut in a single layer over the vegetables in the skillet. Bring to a low simmer. Cover with foil or a lid and place in the oven. Bake until just opaque in the thickest part, 12 to 14 minutes, depending on thickness.

Serve the halibut with the vegetables and pan juices in heated soup plates.

Makes 4 servings

Per serving: 270 calories, 4.5 g fat, 0.5 g saturated fat, 43 g protein, 7 g carbohydrates, 0 g dietary fiber, 65 mg cholesterol, 490 mg sodium

Oven-Steamed Salmon, Hong Kong–Style

Prep: 8 minutes • Cook: 22 minutes

This delicious and very calorie-wise preparation is also wonderful with scallops or shrimp. And it's so versatile that you can prepare it for just one serving; see Dining for One version on the opposite page for cooking times and amounts. If you like, sprinkle each portion with ¼ teaspoon of toasted sesame seeds before serving.

3 tablespoons reduced-sodium soy sauce

2 large garlic cloves, minced

1 tablespoon finely chopped peeled fresh ginger

1 tablespoon medium dry sherry

1½ pounds skinned salmon fillet, cut into four 6-ounce portions

⅛ teaspoon salt

1 bunch scallions, diagonally sliced (about 1 cup)

Preheat oven to 425°F. Set out two rimmed baking sheets.

In a cup, mix the soy sauce, garlic, ginger, and sherry. Tear off four 18-inch-long pieces of heavy-duty foil. Fold each piece of foil crosswise like a book, then open up. Coat one half of each sheet with olive oil cooking spray. In the center of the sprayed half, place a piece of salmon and sprinkle with some salt. Spoon 1 heaping tablespoon of the soy sauce mixture over each piece of salmon and sprinkle with ¼ of the scallions.

Fold the other side of the foil over the food. Crimp the edges tightly to seal. Place the packets on the baking sheets. Bake until the salmon is just opaque in the thickest part, about 20 minutes. Slide the contents of the packets onto warmed dinner plates and serve right away.

Makes 4 servings

Per serving: 330 calories, 19 g fat, 3.5 g saturated fat, 34 g protein, 3 g carbohydrates, 0 g dietary fiber, 100 mg cholesterol, 850 mg sodium

Scallop Variation

Prepare as directed above, using 1½ pounds sea scallops, tough tendons at sides removed, rinsed, and patted dry. Bake for 15 minutes, or until just opaque in the thickest part.

Shrimp Variation

Prepare as directed above, using 1½ pounds peeled and deveined large shrimp. Bake for 15 minutes, or until just opaque in the thickest part.

Dining for One

    2 teaspoons reduced-sodium soy sauce

    1 medium garlic clove, minced

    ¾ teaspoon finely chopped peeled fresh ginger

    ¾ teaspoon medium dry sherry

    One 6-ounce skinned salmon fillet, 6 ounces peeled and deveined shrimp, or 6 ounces sea scallops, tough tendons at sides removed, rinsed, and patted dry

    Pinch salt

    ¼ cup diagonally sliced scallions

Prepare as directed above, using these amounts. Bake for 15 minutes, or until just opaque in the thickest part.

Seafood in Brodo

Prep: 25 minutes • Cook: 25 minutes

In Italian, *brodo* means broth. Here seafood is simmered in a richly flavored broth, giving it succulence without adding fat. Vary the seafood depending on your taste and what looks good in the market. You can make this with all scallops, if that strikes your fancy, or swap littleneck clams for mussels—they'll cook in about the same amount of time. For instructions on cleaning mussels, see page 235.

> 2 cups fat-free reduced-sodium chicken broth
> 1 small onion, halved and thinly sliced
> 3 tablespoons dry white wine
> 1 tablespoon white rice wine vinegar
> 3 garlic cloves, thinly sliced
> 1 sprig fresh thyme or ⅛ teaspoon dried
> 2 cups zucchini (about 1 small to medium zucchini), sliced into
>   thin half-moons
> 1 medium red bell pepper, cut into thin strips, strips cut in half
> 6 ounces peeled and deveined large shrimp, tails left on
> 6 ounces sea scallops, rinsed and patted dry, cut in half through
>   the center, tough tendon at sides removed
> 12 medium mussels, well scrubbed and debearded
> 1 medium plum tomato, diced (about ¼ cup)
> 3 tablespoons chopped fresh Italian parsley

In a wide Dutch oven or large deep skillet, stir the broth, onion, wine, vinegar, garlic, and thyme. Bring to a boil over high heat. Reduce the heat to medium, cover, and simmer for 5 minutes.

Add the zucchini and bell pepper; cover and simmer until tender, about 5 minutes longer. Stir in the shrimp, scallops, and mussels. Cover and cook, stirring occasionally, until the shrimp and scallops are just opaque in the thickest part and the mussels have opened, 4 to 6 minutes.

Remove from the heat and stir in the tomato and parsley. Serve right away in deep bowls.

Makes 4 servings (8 cups)

*Per serving: 170 calories, 2.5 g fat, 0 g saturated fat, 24 g protein,
11 g carbohydrates, 2 g dietary fiber, 90 mg cholesterol, 470 mg sodium*

Roasted Sage-Lemon Salmon

Prep: 4 minutes • Cook: 14 minutes

Silvery-leafed sage—most often thought of as the main flavoring in
Thanksgiving turkey stuffing—has a natural affinity for salmon. This is a
super recipe that goes together in minutes. Any leftovers are terrific cold
for lunch the next day or can be used to prepare Grilled Salmon Salad
(page 218).

> $1\frac{1}{4}$ **pounds skinned salmon fillet, cut in four 5-ounce portions**
>
> **2 tablespoon fresh lemon juice**
>
> **1 teaspoon dried sage, crumbled**
>
> $\frac{3}{4}$ **teaspoon coarsely ground black pepper**
>
> $\frac{1}{2}$ **teaspoon kosher salt**
>
> **Lemon wedges**

Preheat the oven to 450°F. Coat a rimmed baking sheet with olive oil
cooking spray.

Place the salmon on the prepared baking sheet. Drizzle evenly with the
lemon juice. In a cup, mix the sage, pepper, and salt with your fingers.
Sprinkle evenly over the salmon.

Roast the salmon until just opaque in the thickest part, 9 to 12 minutes,
depending on thickness. Transfer to warmed dinner plates and serve
with lemon wedges.

Makes 4 servings

*Per serving: 260 calories, 15 g fat, 3 g saturated fat, 28 g protein,
2 g carbohydrates, 0 g dietary fiber, 85 mg cholesterol, 320 mg sodium*

Seafood Salad Positano

Prep: 20 minutes • Cook: 15 minutes • Standing: 15 minutes or longer

Elegant for a summer dinner on the porch or at the seaside, this is also good cold the next day. It's perfect for company. Serve with steamed asparagus.

1 cup fat-free reduced-sodium chicken broth

⅓ cup dry white wine

2 garlic cloves, minced

¼ teaspoon salt

⅛ to ¼ teaspoon crushed red pepper flakes

10 ounces peeled and deveined large shrimp, tails left on

10 ounces scallops, rinsed and patted dry, tough tendon at sides removed, cut in half crosswise

4 ounces skinned firm whitefish fillet, such as tilapia, tilefish, or halibut, cut in 1-inch chunks

1 cup (4 ounces) crabmeat, picked over

½ cup thinly sliced tender celery hearts

½ cup quartered water-packed canned artichoke hearts, drained

½ cup chopped fresh Italian parsley

½ cup sliced water-packed jarred roasted red peppers, drained

3 tablespoons chopped pitted kalamata olives

2 tablespoons fresh lemon juice

In a large deep skillet, bring the broth, wine, garlic, ⅛ teaspoon salt, and red pepper flakes to a boil over high heat. Reduce the heat to medium, cover, and simmer for 5 minutes to blend the flavors.

Stir in the shrimp, scallops, and fish. Cover and cook, gently stirring often, until the seafood is opaque in the thickest part, 4 to 5 minutes.

Remove from the heat. With a slotted spoon, gently transfer the seafood to a salad bowl, reserving ¼ cup of the cooking liquid. Cover loosely and let cool to lukewarm, about 15 minutes.

Gently fold in the crabmeat, celery, artichoke hearts, parsley, roasted peppers, olives, lemon juice, the reserved cooking liquid, and remaining ⅛ teaspoon salt. Serve immediately or cover and chill to serve later.

Makes 4 servings (4½ cups)

Per serving: 250 calories, 4.5 g fat, 4.5 g saturated fat, 39 g protein, 8 g carbohydrates, 1 g dietary fiber, 170 mg cholesterol, 840 mg sodium

Mussels with Soy and Sherry

Prep: 20 minutes ● Cook: 24 minutes

To clean the mussels, scrub them under cold running water using a stiff brush. Discard any with broken shells or mussels that are open and don't close up when tapped or pressed shut. Pull out the "beard" if it's there; it will be sticking out along the unhinged side. Rinse the mussels again.

> **1 cup fat-free reduced-sodium chicken broth**
>
> **¼ cup medium dry sherry**
>
> **3 garlic cloves, minced**
>
> **1 tablespoon finely chopped peeled fresh ginger**
>
> **1 bunch scallions, thinly sliced**
>
> **2 tablespoons reduced-sodium soy sauce**
>
> **48 medium mussels (about 3 pounds), scrubbed and debearded (see above)**

In a wide Dutch oven or large deep skillet, stir together the broth, sherry, garlic, and ginger. Bring to a boil over high heat.

Reduce the heat to medium, cover, and simmer for 3 minutes. Stir in the scallions and soy sauce; cover and simmer 2 minutes longer.

Add the mussels; stir gently and increase the heat to high. Cover and cook the mussels, shaking the pot and stirring frequently, until the shells are open, about 5 minutes. Remove from the heat and discard any un-opened shells. Spoon the mussels into soup plates, ladling the cooking juices over them. Serve right away.

Makes 4 servings

Per serving: 190 calories, 4.5 g fat, 1 g saturated fat, 24 g protein, 10 g carbohydrates, 0 g dietary fiber, 55 mg cholesterol, 990 mg sodium

Scallop and Vegetable Packets

Prep: 12 minutes ● Cook: 30 minutes

This is a great dish for busy people. In short order the fish and veggies are on the table—with no stirring and no pots to wash! Make this for the family or just for yourself (see Dining for One version on the opposite page).

> **2 packed cups baby spinach**
>
> **2 cups sliced yellow summer squash**
>
> **1 pound sea scallops, rinsed and patted dry, tough tendon at sides removed**
>
> **20 slender asparagus spears, tough ends snapped off, cut in 2-inch lengths (about 2 cups)**
>
> **4 slices sweet onion, rings separated**
>
> **4 slices tomato**
>
> **⅓ cup chopped fresh Italian parsley**
>
> **4 teaspoons vermouth or dry white wine**
>
> **½ teaspoon salt**
>
> **¼ teaspoon freshly ground black pepper**

Preheat the oven to 425°F. Set out two rimmed baking sheets.

Tear off four 20-inch-long sheets of heavy-duty foil. Fold each piece of foil crosswise like a book, then open up. Coat one half of each sheet with olive oil cooking spray.

In the center of each sprayed half, arrange ½ cup spinach, ½ cup squash, ¼ (4 ounces) of the scallops, ½ cup asparagus, 1 slice onion, and 1 slice tomato. Sprinkle with a heaping tablespoon parsley. Drizzle with 1 teaspoon vermouth or wine, and sprinkle with some salt and pepper.

Fold the other side of the foil over the food. Crimp the edges tightly to seal. Place the packets on the baking sheets.

Bake until the scallops are opaque in the thickest part and the vegetables are tender, about 20 minutes.

Transfer the contents of each packet to a heated dinner plate and serve right away.

Makes 4 servings

Per serving: 140 calories, 1 g fat, 0 g saturated fat, 22 g protein, 10 g carbohydrates, 2 g dietary fiber, 35 mg cholesterol, 510 mg sodium

Dining for One

   ½ cup spinach

   ½ cup sliced yellow squash

   4 ounce sea scallops

   5 slender asparagus spears, tough ends snapped off, cut in 2-inch
      lengths

   1 slice sweet onion, rings separated

   1 slice tomato

   1 heaping tablespoon chopped fresh Italian parsley

   1 teaspoon vermouth or dry white wine

   ⅛ teaspoon salt

   Pinch freshly ground black pepper

Prepare as previously directed. Bake until the scallops are opaque in the thickest part and the vegetables are tender, about 20 minutes.

Yucatan-Style Grilled Swordfish

Prep: 6 minutes • Marinate: 15 minutes • Cook: 14 minutes

To provide deep flavor, lime zest, garlic, and aromatic spices are smashed to a paste and spread over the fish before broiling. We loved the fish atop tender baby greens, letting the juices dress and wilt them—adding a spritz of lime juice. You can also make this with mahi mahi or shark.

Note: Swordfish is often sold with the skin on, but the skin is tough and unpleasant and should be removed. Ask the fishmonger to do this, or do it yourself with a sharp knife. Also trim off the dark reddish portions, which can be bitter. Then cut the fish into 7-ounce portions. You'll need to purchase a few ounces more than you need to account for the trimming.

> 1 tablespoon grated lime zest
> 2 large garlic cloves, coarsely chopped
> $1\frac{3}{4}$ teaspoons chili powder
> $\frac{1}{2}$ teaspoon ground cumin
> $\frac{1}{2}$ teaspoon kosher salt
> Pinch ground cinnamon
> 3 tablespoons fresh lime juice
> $1\frac{3}{4}$ pounds 1-inch-thick trimmed swordfish steaks (see note), cut
>   in four 7-ounce portions
> Lime wedges

On a cutting board, finely chop the lime zest and garlic together. Mix in the chili powder, cumin, salt, and cinnamon. Using the flat side of a chef's knife, rub the mixture on the board to form a slightly damp paste. Scrape into a cup and stir in the lime juice.

Put the swordfish on a large plate. Spoon the flavor paste over both sides, spreading it with the back of a spoon. Cover and let stand for 15 minutes.

Meanwhile, place the oven rack as close to the broiler element as possible and preheat the broiler. Coat a broiler-pan rack with olive oil cooking spray.

Place the swordfish on the prepared broiler pan; scrape any flavor paste from the plate on top. Broil until just opaque in the thickest part, 5 to 7 minutes.

Serve hot with lime wedges.

Serves 4

Per serving: 250 calories, 8 g fat, 2 g saturated fat, 40 g protein, 3 g carbohydrates, 0 g dietary fiber, 75 mg cholesterol, 430 mg sodium

Strawberry Soup

Prep: 10 minutes

This refreshing dessert is best freshly made.

> **1 pound fresh strawberries, rinsed and hulled**
> **⅓ cup light sugar-free strawberry preserves**
> **¾ cup plain nonfat yogurt**
> **Pinch ground cinnamon**

Thinly slice enough strawberries to measure 1 cup and reserve. Cut the rest into thick slices.

In a food processor, process the thick-sliced berries and preserves until finely pureed. Add the yogurt and process until smooth.

Transfer to a bowl and stir in the reserved sliced strawberries and cinnamon. Ladle into bowls or mugs and serve.

Makes 4 servings (about 3 cups)

Per serving: 70 calories, 0 g fat, 0 g saturated fat, 3 g protein, 19 g carbohydrates, 2 g dietary fiber, 0 mg cholesterol, 25 mg sodium

Lime-Garlic Grilled Cornish Hens

Prep: 10 minutes • Marinate: at least 2 hours or overnight • Cook: 40 minutes

If you like spicy, use ½ teaspoon crushed red pepper flakes or add a minced chile to the marinade. For deepest flavor, marinate the hens overnight.

2 Cornish game hens, each about 1¼ pounds
⅓ cup fresh lime juice
3 garlic cloves, minced
1½ tablespoons reduced-sodium soy sauce
2 teaspoons grated orange zest
¼ teaspoon crushed red pepper flakes

Cut the wing tips off the hens. With poultry shears, cut down along both sides of the hen's backbone to remove it and discard. Open the hen up and cut it in half down the center of the breast. Repeat with the other hen.

In a measuring cup, stir together the lime juice, garlic, soy sauce, orange zest, and red pepper flakes. Put the hens in a resealable plastic freezer bag; pour in the marinade. Seal the bag and squish it so the marinade coats evenly. Place the bag in a bowl in case of leaks. Marinate the hens in the refrigerator at least 2 hours or overnight.

Heat a barbecue grill to medium. Oil the grill.

Remove the hens from the marinade. Drain the marinade into a small saucepan, bring to a full boil, and boil for 2 minutes.

Place the hens skin side down on the grill. Baste with some marinade. Grill until lightly browned on the underside, about 10 minutes. Use a metal spatula to loosen the hens and turn.

Continue grilling, basting occasionally, and turning and moving as necessary, until no longer pink in the thickest part, 15 to 20 minutes longer. Discard any remaining marinade. Serve the hens, removing the skin before eating.

Makes 4 servings

Per serving: 160 calories, 4.5 g fat, 1 g saturated fat, 26 g protein, 3 g carbohydrates, 0 g dietary fiber, 115 mg cholesterol, 410 mg sodium

Micro-Spice Butternut Squash

Prep: 3 minutes • Cook: 7 minutes

For real convenience, look for packages of diced peeled butternut squash available at some groceries and natural food stores. Otherwise, buy a whole butternut squash and, using a sturdy vegetable peeler, cut and peel what you need. This would be nice topped with a tablespoon of nonfat yogurt. I find that this dish makes a nice complement to fish.

**1 cup 1-inch chunks peeled and seeded butternut squash (about
    5 ounces)**
2 tablespoons water
⅛ teaspoon ground cinnamon
Pinch ground nutmeg
Pinch salt
Pinch freshly ground black pepper

Put the squash chunks in a shallow microwave-safe dish or pie plate. Drizzle with the water and sprinkle with the cinnamon, nutmeg, salt, and pepper. Toss to mix.

Cover with waxed paper or vented plastic wrap and microwave on High until the squash is tender, 5 to 6 minutes. Let stand a few minutes before serving, as the squash will be very hot.

Makes 1 serving (about 1 cup)

*Per serving: 70 calories, 0 g fat, 0 g saturated fat, 1 g protein,
17 g carbohydrates, 3 g dietary fiber, 0 mg cholesterol, 150 mg sodium*

THE CONTINUING PLAN

If you want to continue on the diet for more than 10 days or would prefer to lose weight at a slower pace, I suggest that you switch to B-list foods, which offer greater variety in your food and dining choices and a slight increase in your daily caloric intake. During this period, it's natural for your weight loss to slow somewhat after the significant loss of the 10-Day TurboCharge Diet with the addition of the extra calories. Those who tend to lose weight slowly or don't want additional variety may, with their physician's approval, remain on the A-list eating plan. It's recommended, however, for nutritional balance that at least one of your allowed snacks consist of a fruit unless you're one of those rare people for whom fruit is an appetite trigger.

The B-list introduces more complex carbohydrates and gourmet choices, some of which may be somewhat higher in calories and have slightly more fat than the A-list meals. For breakfast, if you don't have a history of overeating cereal *and* you're willing to measure out a *single* serving (I've observed that most people tend to use two to three times that amount), you may select a cereal. However, I've found that people who have trouble losing weight or are very "carbohydrate sensitive," i.e., carbohydrates increase their appetite, may benefit more from continuing with a protein breakfast. If you would like to add a cereal, a favorite breakfast is my Cinnamon 'n Berries recipe (page 246). Whatever you decide, don't be fooled into believing that by selecting a "healthy cereal," you're doing something wonderful for your waistline. Most healthy cereals are myths. If a cereal doesn't have double-digit fiber and single-digit sugar grams per serving, it's probably not worth your time. Also, sugar-coated cereals or those containing dried fruits or nuts tend to be very high on the "abuse scale" and often equally high in calories. It's best to avoid them and all cereals that are more than 120 calories a serving. A high-fiber, no-sugar-added oatmeal is another option. But be sure to pass on the instant varieties, because they tend to have less fiber.

While I've tried to eliminate many of the foods on the ABC Eating Plan that I've noticed caused dieters to lose control most often, you might want to exercise some caution when choosing some of the meals on this phase of the diet, particularly if you run across one that contains a food you have a history of abusing. This is especially true of any meals containing bread and bread products. I've noted that whenever someone reintroduces bread into their diet—especially at breakfast—they quickly get used to having bread at meals, and it can lead to greater quantities.

On the other hand, I've found that some people don't seem to associate English muffins with bread abuse, and they may ultimately prove to be a better choice if you're trying to Box In a bread product. If a light English muffin is not available at your supermarket, try half a regular English muffin (particularly if you lose weight slowly). Always look for the highest-fiber English muffin available.

In the B-list, I also introduce you to the VitaMuffin—the only muffin I recommend at 100 calories for 2 ounces, or 200 calories for 4 ounces. For some people, muffins, like bread, are a bridge back into the realm of baked goods. Or, they may associate the VitaMuffin with other "light" muffins, which are often not light at all and frequently contain dozens of unwanted calories and grams of fat and/or sugar. I've found that people who get used to eating a muffin for breakfast are more likely to switch to a regular muffin when this one is not available, which could cause problems. Once again, if this scenario does not apply to your history, I don't have a problem with you having an occasional VitaMuffin.

I do want to reiterate one other point. If baked goods are not a problem for you, as they're not for some of my clients, you shouldn't feel inclined to give them up. But from a caloric and nutritional point of view, they're a group of foods that should be used sparingly.

The B-list introduces several new meat dishes, including some made with veal and lamb, which were verboten during the 10-Day TurboCharge Diet. If you choose veal or lamb, I suggest loin, lamb chops, medallions (without the fat), and eye of the round (which tends to be the lowest in calories). All meats, including beef and pork, can be increased to 4 ounces per meal and two servings a week for women, and 6 ounces per meal and three servings a week for men. You should be aware that some cuts of meat, especially sirloin and filet mignon, have a slight edge in calories. So, if you decide on a meat dish from the menu, for example Chef Miriam's Pan-Grilled Beef Tenderloin and Vegetables Oreganata, try to prepare it with one of the brands I recommend. Many of my clients like Laura's Lean Beef products. Ostrich and bison are also popular choices that give you the taste and texture of beef but have fewer calories and fat.

If you like pasta, you can have a fixed amount in the form of a frozen entrée such as Stouffers Lean Cuisine Grilled Chicken Caesar (240 calories) or Chicken Carbonara (260 calories). I would *strongly prefer* that you save pasta for the maintenance phase of the eating plan because it's an easy food to abuse in terms of quantity, and it's not a nutritional winner. But if you feel you must have it in this phase, the Stouffers entrées are a good bet, especially since they all come with a protein. Otherwise, use a single serving only of a lower-starch variety such as Carbfit or DeBole's or a whole wheat pasta.

For those of you who enjoy alcohol, I have no problem with you having an occasional drink, preferably dry red or white wine, scotch, or vodka. You should avoid mixed drinks made with juices, regular soda, tonic water (unless diet), or added sugar. It's also a good idea to stay away from relatively benign-looking drinks like martinis, which have more than 350 calories per 3½ ounces. Women can have two or three drinks a week; men can have three or four.

In the second phase of the diet, women can continue to have two snacks a day and men can have three. A dessert for those so inclined might be a cappuccino with fat-free milk, a bag of Knight's Light Popcorn, or a Patisserie de France Orange or Lemon Giurees. If you're having a tough time deciding, simply refer to the snack, dessert, and minimeal menu (page 251) or look through the shopping lists (page 297) until you find something that suits your palate. Once again, avoid any choice you have a history of abusing.

There may be times during this phase of the eating plan that you overindulge or forget to "Box Out" a certain food. You might, for example, have a big piece of lasagna at a holiday party, eat a big Thanksgiving dinner, enjoy a slice of high-calorie birthday cake, or add too much olive oil to your salad while on a vacation in Italy. *Undoubtedly, there will also be times when life events cause you to gain back some of the pounds you've lost or reach a plateau in your weight loss. If that happens, you should simply return to the 10-Day TurboCharge Diet.* The ABC Eating Plan is designed with your life in mind and allows for just such possibilities.

PHASE B:
The Continuing Plan

These items may be enjoyed every day and take 15 or fewer minutes to pre-pare. They are designed to keep your weight loss in the healthy range of 1 to 2 pounds per week. They are not for accelerated weight loss.

Note on suggested serving size: When two amounts are indicated, the lower amount applies to women and the higher amount to men.

Note on high-fiber crackers: My first choice is the GG Scandinavian Bran Crispbread, since it is the only thick cracker with a mere 16 calories, 3 grams of appetite-quenching fiber, and 3 grams of carbohydrates (0 net carbs!). If you are waiting for a shipment to arrive at your local health food store or from the sources indicated in our reference section, you may temporarily substitute the Bran-a-Crisp, WASA Light Rye, FiberRich, or any other thick high-fiber cracker that has no more than 25 calories and at least 2 grams of fiber. All of these crackers have more calories and carbohydrates and less fiber, so I strongly recommend only the GGs.

Note on light cheese: My top choice of a light cheese is Laughing Cow Light, since it comes premeasured in individually wrapped triangles (each of which is only 35 calories). If you can't find Laughing Cow Light, tem-porarily use regular Laughing Cow, since it is only 15 more calories, until you obtain the light ones from the source indicated in our reference sec-tion, or use 2 tablespoons of Alouette Cheese Spread for each Laughing Cow Light or 1 Mini Bonbel Light or Swiss Knight Light. But I strongly recommend Laughing Cow Light because it is the lowest in calories and it is instantly spreadable. Remember: Laughing Cow is wrapped and can travel with you anywhere.

Breakfast Menu

Quick and Easy Breakfast

While these choices are a regular part of my program, the best breakfasts for optimal weight loss and hunger control are still the protein breakfasts of dairy, eggs, GG Bran Crispbread with melted cheese, etc., as in Phase A.

Awesome Oatmeal

Mix ⅓ to ½ cup of dry oatmeal with approximately ½ cup of water. Top with 1 teaspoon cinnamon, 2 tablespoons Walden Farms Calorie Free Fruit Preserves, or 4 to 5 sliced strawberries or 2 tablespoons of blueberries.

Cinnamon 'n Berries

Serve ½ to ¾ cup of Kellogg's All Bran with Extra Fiber, Fiber One, or similar unsweetened bran cereal (cereal must be measured) with not more than ¾ cup of fat-free milk. The cereal choices do not include Raisin Bran. For added flavor, sprinkle with a teaspoon of cinnamon. Top with berries.

Eggs 'n English

Follow the same guidelines for the Omelet Supreme (page 203) or prepare 1 or 2 poached or soft-boiled eggs with one light English muffin (60–80 calories), such as Thomas's. If you don't like English muffins, you can substitute 1 slice of Wonder Light Wheat or Beefsteak Light Rye. For added taste, use a tablespoon of fat-free cream cheese or a few sprays of I Can't Believe It's Not Butter spray on the bread. (This is not for those with a history of abusing breads.)

Gourmet Breakfast

These special choices are to be used one to three times a week, especially on weekends.

Belgian Supreme

Prepare with 2 Van's 7-Grain Belgian Waffles, Van's Carb-Manager Waffles, or any multigrain waffle that's 100 calories or less. For added flavor try ½ teaspoon of cinnamon, Splenda, and a few sprays of I Can't Believe It's Not Butter spray.

Gourmet Omelet

Prepare with the same ingredients as the cheese veggie omelet (page 205). For the vegetables, try ½ cup of onions, mushrooms, or broccoli. And select one of the following: 2 ounces of smoked salmon, 2 slices of Butterball Thin 'n Crispy Turkey Bacon, 1 or 2 Armour Lite Breakfast Sausages, or 2 Boca Breakfast Links, or omit the cheese and have

Top Choice for accelerated weight loss

a veggie omelet with 1 Boca Italian Breakfast Sausage.

Waffles 'n Omelet

One Van's 7-Grain Waffle, Van's Carb-Manager Waffles, or any multigrain waffle that's 100 calories or less, with 1 fresh egg and 2 egg whites or 4 ounces egg substitute, mixed with 2 cups of steamed, low-carb, cut-up green and white vegetables.

Eggs 'n Pancakes

Prepare with 1 fresh egg and 2 to 3 eggs whites or 4 ounces of egg substitute and 2 or 3 Aunt Jemima Light Pancakes. You may top the pancakes with 3 or 4 cut strawberries and ½ teaspoon of cinnamon or a small amount of Country Cottage Light Syrup (20 calories) or Walden Farms syrup.

Dr. G.'s Cinnamon French Toast

Imagine a delicious French toast for a mere 100 calories for two pieces: Mix 3 egg whites or 4 ounces of egg substitute with ½ cup of fat-free milk. Beat well. Dip 2 pieces of Wonder Light Whole Wheat Bread into the egg mixture. Put into a frying pan heated over low-to-medium flame until lightly browned on each side. Top with ½ teaspoon cinnamon and Splenda or a drizzle of Country Cottage sugar-free syrup and cinnamon.

On-the-Go Breakfast

Try these delicious choices when you're on the run and don't have time for a sit-down meal.

Muffin 'n Yogurt

Enjoy a VitaMuffin (100 calories only) (page 243) with 4 to 6 ounces of fat-free or low-fat yogurt (Fage Total, Le Carb, Dannon Carb Control, Atkins Yogurt). If you don't want the yogurt, try substituting 1 or 2 Laughing Cow Light Cheese wedges or a hard-cooked egg. This muffin is not recommended for those who have a history of abusing muffins or who will switch to regular or light muffins when Vita-Muffins aren't available.

Fast-Food Breakfast

Subway's Vegetable and Egg Omelet

Has 210 calories in a 174-gram serving.

Lunch Menu

Quick and Easy Lunch

These items may be enjoyed every day.

Heavenly Roll

A 6- to 8-piece sushi roll (avoid tempura, spicy sushi, and avocado) is a delicious and healthy way to add a little variety to your lunch menu. Serve with wasabi mustard and a light soy sauce. Add a bowl of miso soup. Women can have this two or three times a week and men daily (it's high in sodium).

Potato Express

Bake 1 white or sweet potato, and melt 1 slice of my recommended fat-free cheese. Add 2 servings of steamed low carb green and white vegetables and a salad. Women should have a small baked potato one or two times a week, and men may have a medium potato three times a week.

Athens Afternoon

This light Greek salad can be made with lettuce, green and red peppers, 5 black olives, oregano, and pepper. Add 3 or 4 ounces of President's Fat-Free Feta Cheese. Do not add grape leaves, and do not order Greek salads in restaurants while on Phases A or B.

Soup 'n Crackers

Health Valley or Tabatchnick Soups with 2 GG crackers or similar high-fiber crackers. The soups can be any selection that is 70 to 100 calories per serving, and you can have 2 servings. Add a salad with nonfat dressing or flavored balsamic vinaigrette and steamed vegetables.

Gourmet Lunch

These special choices are to be used one to three times a week, especially on weekends.

Solar Harvest's Chicken Fajitas

See recipe, page 264.

Frozen Lunch Entrée

Choose any frozen entrée that's a maximum of 250 calories or Amy's brand Shepherd's or Mexican Pot Pie. Serve with 2 cups of steamed low-carb green and white mixed vegetables or a tossed salad. Amy's entrees are in the 150- to 170-calorie range. Do not eat regular shepherd's pie while losing weight.

Seafood Salad Positano

See recipe, page 234.

*Top Choice for accelerated weight loss

On-the-Go Lunch

Try these delicious choices when you're on the run and don't have time for a sit-down meal.

Subway

My top pick is their salads with sliced turkey. If you don't abuse rolls, best bets include the "7-Under-6" sandwich with turkey, lettuce, tomato, and mustard. Women who lose weight slowly may want to have half a roll or the turkey on a salad.

Atkins Bar
(approximately 225 calories)

Light Sandwich Menu

Have with salad with nonfat dressing or flavored balsamic vinaigrette and steamed vegetables or 1 cup of Health Valley or Tabatchnick's soup (70 to 80 calories)

Note: Sandwiches are not for those seeking to avoid bread. If this applies to you, use the GG crackers in lieu of bread (2 GGs equal 1 slice of light bread), or roll the cold cuts in lettuce leaves.

BLT

4 to 6 slices of Butterball Thin 'n Crispy turkey bacon on 2 slices of toasted Wonder Light Whole Wheat topped with Kraft Fat-Free Mayonnaise, lettuce, and 2 slices of tomato.

Ham 'n Cheese on Rye

2 to 4 slices of light ham and 2 or 3 slices of fat-free American cheese (Kraft, Borden's, Weight Watchers) melted over the ham on Beefsteak Light Rye Bread.

Cold Cut Mix

3 or 4 ounces of white meat chicken or turkey or 6 to 8 slices of any light cold cut (10 to 15 calories per slice) on 2 slices of Wonder Light Whole Wheat or Beefsteak Light Rye. (Both of these breads are a mere 10 calories per slice.)

Deli on Rye

4 or 5 slices of Hebrew National Lean Salami or 5 to 7 slices of Hillshire Farms Light Pastrami (a mere 10 calories per slice) on 2 slices of Beefsteak Light.

Dinner Menu

Quick and Easy Dinner

These items may be enjoyed every day.

Hot and Spicy Kabobs

Start with 4 to 6 ounces of turkey, beef, or pork. Cut the meat into medallions, and put onto skewers with mushroom caps, baby onions, cherry tomatoes, and green peppers. Baste with Walden Farms Thick N Spicy Barbecue Sauce.

Chef Miriam's Baked Quesadilla

See recipe, page 252.

A Better Burger

Start with a 4- to 6-ounce white meat turkey burger. Serve with a small baked potato and 1 cup of steamed vegetables and a salad made with nonfat dressing or flavored balsamic vinaigrette. Women can have 1 or 2 small baked potatoes a week; men can have a maximum of 3 small/medium potatoes per week. Do not order turkey burgers in restaurants, because they contain dark meat and skin and are higher in calories than burgers made from white meat.

Solar Harvest's Blueberry Bison (or Lean Beef) Burger with Baked Yam Wedges

See recipe, page 268. Women can have once a week. But fish, chicken, and pork are preferable, particularly fish, if you tend to lose weight slowly.

✳ *Top Choice for accelerated weight loss*

Grilled Veal Scallops with Olive-Artichoke Relish

See recipe, page 257. Women can have once a week. But fish, chicken, and pork are preferable, if you tend to be a slow weight loser.

Solar Harvest's Steak Fajitas

See recipe, page 264.
Women can have once a week. But fish, chicken, and pork are preferable, if you tend to be a slow weight loser.

Crunchy Roll

Two sushi rolls (preferably made with salmon, tuna, or shrimp) lightly sprinkled with tempura flakes. Serve with a medium salad with nonfat dressing or flavored balsamic vinaigrette or a cup of miso soup. Women can have once per week, or they can have sashimi without the rice or cucumber sashimi as often as desired.

Chef Miriam's Recipes

Curried Chicken Breast with Mango Chutney

See recipe, page 256.

Savory Stuffed Chicken Breasts

See recipe, page 266.

Pork Scaloppini with Arugula-Orange Salad

See recipe, page 262.

Snacks and Minimeals

You may select one of these snacks in place of—not in addition to—the snacks on Phase A. These items should be added only after you reach the second phase of the eating plan, i.e., after you've completed 10 days on the TurboCharge Diet. If you tend to lose weight at a slow rate, you may elect to delay adding any of these snacks, or you may omit them entirely, with one exception: For nutritional purposes, it is helpful to have at least one fruit per day.

Van's 7-Grain Belgian Waffles
Enjoy 1 plain waffle or make into Dr. G's Strawberry Shortcake (see recipe on page 85).

Hormel Turkey Pepperoni or Turkey/Beef Jerky (80 calories)

Fresh Fruit
You may choose an apple, pear, nectarine, orange, tangerine, or ½ to 1 small banana.

Skinny Cow Fat-Free Fudge Bars (100 calories each)

Klondike or Carb-Smart Frozen Chocolate Pops (100 calories each)

Knight's or Orville Redenbacher's Light Popcorn (individual bags only)
For optimal weight loss, women should not have this more than twice per week.

Chocolate-Covered Banana
Cut a small banana horizontally, and use only half. Put on a piece of aluminum foil, and cover with Walden Farms Calorie-Free Chocolate Dip. Wrap, and freeze.

Chef Miriam's Amazing Lemony Soup with Crab and Vegetables
See recipe, page 214.

Chef Miriam's Strawberry Soup
See recipe, page 239.

GGs with Cheese and Fruit
See recipe, page 253.

Dr. G.'s Cinnamon French Toast
See recipe, page 247.

Cappuccino and Whipped Cream
Make with Reddi-wip fat-free or light whipped cream.

Gayle's Chocolate Truffles
2 or 3 truffles (30 calories each) for occasional use only

Pria Bar (a chocolate protein bar)

Dilled Cucumber and Yogurt Soup
See recipe, page 215.

Apple Betty
See recipe, page 270.

Patisserie de France Giurees

Chef Miriam's Cinnamon-Pear Crumble
See recipe, page 270.

Baked Quesadilla

Prep: 5 to 7 minutes • Cook: 17 minutes

Look for Mi Pueblito flour tortillas at your supermarket. They're the lowest in calories (80 each) that I've found. If they aren't available, try Buena Vida fat-free flour tortillas, weighing in at 100 calories per tortilla. We used Cabot 50% Light Jalapeno Cheddar (70 calories per ounce), which added lots of flavor.

One 8-inch flour tortilla

¾ cup sliced cremini or white button mushrooms (use presliced)

¾ cup zucchini, sliced in thin half-moons

½ cup short, thin red bell pepper strips

⅓ cup thinly sliced sweet white onion

½ teaspoon chili powder

⅛ teaspoon salt

¼ cup shredded reduced-fat jalapeño Cheddar cheese (see above)

½ cup shredded iceberg lettuce (from a bag)

1 or 2 tablespoons salsa

Preheat the oven to 425°F. Coat a rimmed baking sheet with olive oil cooking spray. Place the tortilla on the baking sheet.

In a medium bowl, mix the mushrooms, zucchini, bell pepper, onion, chili powder, and salt. Mound on the tortilla and sprinkle with the cheese. Cover the pan with foil.

Bake until the vegetables are heated and tender and the cheese has melted, about 15 minutes. Transfer to a plate and top with the shredded lettuce and salsa.

Makes 1 serving

Per serving: 170 calories, 4 g fat, 1 g saturated fat, 9 g protein, 29 g carbohydrates, 5 g dietary fiber, 0 mg cholesterol, 420 mg sodium

GGs with Cheese and Fruit

Prep: 8 minutes

If strawberries and blueberries aren't in season, you can make this spread with chopped apple and/or pear. Enjoy with a cup of tea for a soothing and satisfying snack.

$\frac{1}{4}$ **cup fat-free ricotta cheese**

$\frac{1}{4}$ **cup chopped fresh strawberries**

2 tablespoons chopped fresh blueberries

Pinch ground cinnamon

1 teaspoon light sugar-free strawberry preserves

3 GG Scandinavian Bran Crispbreads

In a small bowl, mix the ricotta, strawberries, blueberries, and cinnamon. Spread evenly over the crispbreads. Top each with some jam and serve.

Makes 1 serving

Per serving: 130 calories, 0 g fat, 0 g saturated fat, 8 g protein, 25 g carbohydrates, 10 g dietary fiber, 10 mg cholesterol, 65 mg sodium

GG Veggie-Cheese Crunch

Prep: 4 minutes

Vary the veggies to suit your taste.

$\frac{1}{4}$ **cup fat-free ricotta cheese**

$\frac{1}{4}$ **cup chopped cucumber**

2 tablespoons chopped red or green bell pepper

1 tablespoon thinly sliced scallion

Salt and freshly ground black pepper, to taste

3 GG Scandinavian Bran Crispbreads

1 tablespoon chopped fresh tomato

In a small bowl, mix the ricotta, cucumber, bell pepper, and scallion. Season to taste with salt and pepper. Spread evenly over the crispbreads. Top each with some tomato and serve.

Makes 1 serving (about $\frac{1}{2}$ cup spread)

Per serving: 110 calories, 0 g fat, 0 g saturated fat, 9 g protein, 17 g carbohydrates, 10 g dietary fiber, 10 mg cholesterol, 210 mg sodium

Broiled Lamb Chops
with Black Pepper and Herbs

Prep: 5 minutes ● Cook: 16 minutes

A perfect way to start this meal is with steamed fresh artichokes. Instead of butter, use fresh lemon wedges. If fresh artichokes aren't in season, frozen artichoke hearts are good, too. Cook according to package directions and flavor them with chopped fresh parsley, chopped chives or scallions, and a squeeze of lemon.

See the Dining for One version on the opposite page.

2 garlic cloves, minced

1 teaspoon dried sage, crumbled

½ teaspoon dried oregano

½ teaspoon kosher salt

½ teaspoon coarsely ground black pepper

Four 6-ounce bone-in, well-trimmed loin lamb chops

Lemon wedges

Preheat the broiler. Spray a broiler-pan rack with olive oil cooking spray.

In a cup, mix the garlic, herbs, salt, and pepper. Press onto both sides of the chops. Broil 4 to 6 inches from the heat, turning once, 12 to 14 minutes (depending on thickness), for medium.

Serve with lemon wedges.

Makes 4 servings

Per serving: 100 calories, 4 g fat, 1.5 g saturated fat, 14 g protein, 2 g carbohydrates, 0 g dietary fiber, 45 mg cholesterol, 280 mg sodium

Dining for One
  1 small minced garlic clove
  $\frac{1}{4}$ teaspoon dried sage
  $\frac{1}{8}$ teaspoon dried oregano
  $\frac{1}{8}$ teaspoon kosher salt
  $\frac{1}{8}$ teaspoon coarsely ground black pepper
  1 6-ounce, bone-in, trimmed loin lamb chop

In a cup, mix garlic, sage, oregano, salt, and pepper. Rub over both sides of the lamb chop. Broil as above. Serve with a lemon wedge.

Curried Chicken Breast with Mango Chutney

Prep: 5 minutes • Broil: 10 minutes

If ripe mango isn't available, use papaya or cantaloupe. Serve with steamed green beans and zucchini.

For the chutney:

$\frac{1}{2}$ **cup diced ripe mango**

$\frac{1}{4}$ **cup chopped red bell pepper**

$\frac{1}{4}$ **cup chopped hothouse cucumber**

2 tablespoons plain nonfat yogurt

1 tablespoon chopped sweet red or white onion

$\frac{1}{8}$ **teaspoon curry powder**

For the chicken:

1 teaspoon curry powder

$\frac{1}{2}$ **teaspoon salt**

$\frac{1}{4}$ **teaspoon freshly ground black pepper**

Four 5-ounce skinless, boneless chicken breast halves

To make the chutney: In a small bowl, stir together the mango, bell pepper, cucumber, yogurt, onion, and curry powder. Set aside while cooking the chicken.

To make the chicken: Preheat the broiler. Coat a broiler-pan rack with olive oil cooking spray.

In a cup, mix the curry powder, salt, and pepper. Sprinkle evenly over both sides of the chicken, rubbing it in with your fingers. Place the chicken on the prepared broiler pan.

Broil the chicken 3 to 5 inches from the heat until lightly golden and no longer pink in the center, 8 to 10 minutes. Remove from the heat.

Serve the chicken with the mango chutney.

Makes 4 servings (scant 1 cup chutney)

Per serving: 180 calories, 2 g fat, 0.5 g saturated fat, 33 g protein, 5 g carbohydrates, 0 g dietary fiber, 80 mg cholesterol, 390 mg sodium

Grilled Veal Scallops
with Olive-Artichoke Relish

Prep: 10 minutes • Cook: 15 minutes

If you prefer, you can make this with thin-sliced turkey or chicken cutlets or with thin boneless pork chops. It's good served at room temperature, and the relish may be made an hour or so ahead of time.

For the relish:

> 1 cup coarsely chopped water-packed canned artichoke hearts, drained
>
> $\frac{1}{2}$ cup coarsely chopped jarred roasted red peppers, drained
>
> 3 tablespoons chopped pitted kalamata olives
>
> 2 tablespoons chopped red onion
>
> 1 tablespoon fresh lemon juice

For the veal:

> 1 to $1\frac{1}{4}$ pounds thin veal scallops
>
> 1 teaspoon dried thyme, crumbled
>
> $\frac{1}{2}$ teaspoon salt
>
> $\frac{1}{4}$ teaspoon freshly ground black pepper
>
> Lemon wedges for serving

For the relish: In a medium bowl, mix the artichoke hearts, roasted peppers, olives, onion, and lemon juice.

For the veal: Place a veal scallop on a cutting board and cover with a sheet of plastic wrap. Pound with a meat mallet or the bottom of a heavy pot to an $\frac{1}{8}$ inch thickness. Repeat with the remaining veal.

Sprinkle the veal on both sides with thyme, salt, and pepper.

Coat a nonstick grill pan with olive oil cooking spray. Heat over medium heat for 3 minutes. Add half the veal and cook about 2 minutes, until browned on the underside. Turn and cook about 1 minute longer, until browned but just a little pink in the thickest part. Transfer to a warmed platter, and cover loosely to keep warm. Repeat with the remaining veal.

Serve the veal with the artichoke relish and lemon wedges.

Makes 4 servings ($1\frac{3}{4}$ cups artichoke relish)

Per serving: 280 calories, 18 g fat, 7 g saturated fat, 22 g protein, 7 g carbohydrates, 2 g dietary fiber, 80 mg cholesterol, 710 mg sodium

Grilled Spice-Rubbed Pork Tenderloin with Cucumber-Yogurt Sauce

Prep: 5 minutes • Cook: 30 minutes

Pork tenderloin is an overlooked cut of meat. It's tender, flavorful, and especially juicy if it's cooked to a turn (ideally 155°F). Tenderloins generally come in packages of two; trim and freeze the other piece for another meal.

For the pork:

> **2 teaspoons ground cumin**
>
> **1 teaspoon ground coriander**
>
> **1 teaspoon paprika**
>
> **$\frac{1}{2}$ teaspoon kosher salt**
>
> **$\frac{1}{2}$ teaspoon freshly ground black pepper**
>
> **$\frac{1}{4}$ teaspoon garlic powder**
>
> **One $1\frac{1}{4}$-pound trimmed pork tenderloin**

For the sauce:

> **$\frac{1}{2}$ cup shredded hothouse cucumber**
>
> **$\frac{3}{4}$ cup plain nonfat yogurt**
>
> **1 small garlic clove, crushed through a press**
>
> **$\frac{1}{4}$ teaspoon kosher salt**
>
> **Pinch cayenne pepper**

Heat a barbecue grill to medium. Oil the grill.

To make the pork: In a cup, mix the cumin, coriander, paprika, salt, pepper, and garlic powder. Place the pork on a sheet of foil. Coat lightly with olive oil cooking spray. Sprinkle the spices over the pork, rolling the pork, and rubbing them into the surface.

Grill the pork, turning often, until browned on the outside and an instant-read thermometer inserted in the center registers 155°F, 20 to 25 minutes. Transfer to a platter and let stand while preparing the sauce.

To make the sauce: Put the cucumber in a small strainer and press down with a spoon to squeeze out excess liquid. Transfer to a medium bowl and stir in the yogurt, garlic, salt, and cayenne pepper.

Slice the pork and serve with the sauce.

Makes 4 servings (1 cup sauce)

Per serving: 200 calories, 5 g fat, 1.5 g saturated fat, 32 g protein, 5 g carbohydrates, 1 g dietary fiber, 95 mg cholesterol, 450 mg sodium

Pan-Grilled Beef Tenderloin and Vegetables Oreganata

Prep: 15 minutes • Cook: 25 minutes

A ridged grill pan with a nonstick coating is an indispensable low-cal cooking tool, especially for those who don't have an outdoor grill. It imparts plenty of grilled flavor—without using fat. This dish can also be made with boneless beef top loin steaks. They're thinner and will cook a bit more quickly.

3 or 4 garlic cloves, minced

2 tablespoons chopped fresh Italian parsley

$\frac{3}{4}$ teaspoon dried oregano

$\frac{3}{4}$ teaspoon kosher salt

$\frac{1}{2}$ teaspoon freshly ground black pepper

$\frac{1}{8}$ teaspoon crushed red pepper flakes

$1\frac{1}{4}$ pounds well-trimmed beef tenderloin, cut into four 5-ounce portions

1 package (6 ounces) sliced portabello mushrooms

1 large red bell pepper, cut into $\frac{1}{2}$-inch strips

1 sweet white onion, halved and cut into thick slices

1 tablespoon balsamic vinegar

In a cup, with a spoon, mix the garlic, parsley, oregano, salt, black pepper, and red pepper flakes.

Flatten the tenderloin slices to a 1-inch thickness with your hand so they cook evenly. Rub each with 2 tablespoons garlic mixture, pressing it onto both sides.

Put the vegetables in a bowl. Add the remaining garlic mixture and the balsamic vinegar and toss to coat.

Coat a grill pan with olive oil cooking spray. Heat over medium heat for 3 minutes. Add the tenderloin slices and pan-grill 4 to 6 minutes per side for medium-rare. Transfer to a warmed platter and cover loosely to keep warm.

Meanwhile, coat a large nonstick skillet with olive oil cooking spray. Heat over medium heat for 1 minute. Add the vegetables and cook, stirring often, until tender and lightly charred, about 10 minutes. If pan starts to scorch, add a tablespoon of water, repeating if necessary.

Spoon the vegetables onto the platter next to the beef and serve immediately.

Makes 4 servings

Per serving: 200 calories, 5 g fat, 2 g saturated fat, 30 g protein, 10 g carbohydrates, 1 g dietary fiber, 75 mg cholesterol, 430 mg sodium

Mustard-Crumbed Chicken

Prep: 8 minutes • Cook: 22 minutes

Good with steamed vegetables. Try a colorful and healthful assortment including carrots, turnips, green beans, and red peppers.

1 tablespoon grainy mustard

1 tablespoon plain nonfat yogurt

¼ teaspoon poultry seasoning

One 4-ounce skinless boneless chicken-breast half

3 GG Bran Crispbreads, crumbled, put in a resealable plastic freezer bag, and crushed fine with a rolling pin (about ¼ cup)

Preheat the oven to 375°F. Coat a small baking pan with olive oil cooking spray.

In a small shallow bowl, mix the mustard, yogurt, and seasoning. Turn the chicken in the mixture to coat both sides. Put the crumbs on a sheet of waxed paper and roll the chicken in the crumbs.

Transfer to the prepared baking pan. Mist the chicken with olive oil cooking spray. Bake until the chicken is no longer pink in the thickest part, 15 to 17 minutes.

Serve hot.

Makes 1 serving

Per serving: 230 calories, 3 g fat, 0.5 g saturated fat, 30 g protein, 18 g carbohydrates, 3 g dietary fiber, 65 mg cholesterol, 440 mg sodium

Pork Scaloppini
with Arugula-Orange Salad

Prep: 6 minutes • Cook: 22 minutes

Not in the mood for pork? Simply prepare this with thin-sliced chicken or turkey breast cutlets. If arugula is not available, substitute baby spinach.

For the salad:

1 medium navel orange

1 tablespoon orange juice

1 tablespoon balsamic vinegar

1 teaspoon extra-virgin olive oil

$\frac{1}{8}$ teaspoon salt

$\frac{1}{4}$ cup thinly sliced sweet white onion

4 cups arugula, rinsed and spun dry

1 Belgian endive, thinly sliced

For the pork:

$1\frac{1}{4}$ pounds thin boneless pork loin chops, well trimmed

1 teaspoon grated orange zest (from orange in salad)

1 teaspoon dried marjoram

$\frac{1}{2}$ teaspoon salt

$\frac{1}{4}$ teaspoon crushed red pepper flakes

To make the salad: Grate 1 teaspoon zest from the orange and reserve for the pork. With a sharp or serrated knife, cut the peel and white pith off the orange. Cut the orange in half through the stem end, place the halves flat on a cutting board, and slice.

In a salad bowl, mix the orange juice, balsamic vinegar, olive oil, and salt with a fork. Add the orange slices and onion to the dressing; place the arugula and Belgian endive on top. Don't toss yet.

To make the pork: Place a pork chop on a cutting board and cover with a sheet of plastic wrap. Pound with a meat mallet or the bottom of a heavy pot to an $\frac{1}{8}$-inch thickness. Repeat with the remaining pork.

Preheat the broiler. Coat a broiler-pan rack with olive oil cooking spray.

In a cup, with your fingers, mix the reserved orange zest, marjoram, salt, and crushed red pepper. Rub the mixture over both sides of the pork.

Arrange the pork in a single layer on the prepared broiler pan. Broil 3 or 4 inches from the heat until lightly browned and no longer pink in the center, 5 to 7 minutes. Transfer the pork to a plate.

Toss the salad. Divide onto four dinner plates and place ¼ of the pork on each.

Makes 4 servings (5 cups salad)

Per serving: 210 calories, 4.5 g fat, 1 g saturated fat, 33 g protein,
8 g carbohydrates, 2 g dietary fiber, 80 mg cholesterol, 630 mg sodium

Chicken or Steak Fajitas

Prep: 2½ hours (includes 2 hours for marinating) ● **Cook: 25 minutes**

This is a great recipe that will impress dinner guests but doesn't take a lot of preparation. Just be sure to leave enough time for the meat to marinate to guarantee the flavor and juiciness.

½ cup lime juice

2 tablespoons cilantro, chopped

1 pound lean steak, cut into strips, or 1 pound boneless, skinless chicken breasts, cut into strips

4 whole wheat tortillas

1 tablespoon olive oil

1 large onion, cut into strips

1 large green pepper, cut into strips

2 teaspoons cumin

1 teaspoon chile powder

2 teaspoons garlic powder

Guacamole, salsa or pico de gallo

Combine the lime juice and cilantro in a nonreactive bowl. Add the meat strips and marinate in the refrigerator for 2 to 4 hours. Warm the tortillas in the oven.

Heat the oil in a skillet over medium heat. Add the onion and sauté until translucent. Add the peppers and sauté for 2 more minutes. Add the strips of meat along with the marinade and continue to sauté, stirring only occasionally, until meat is almost cooked through.

Season the whole skillet with cumin, chile powder, and garlic powder. Sauté for 1 more minute. Remove skillet from heat and serve meat with the warmed tortillas, guacamole, and salsa.

Makes 4 servings

Per serving: 340 calories, 8 g fat, 1 g saturated fat, 32 g protein, 32 g carbohydrates, 4 g dietary fiber, 65 mg cholesterol, 260 mg sodium

Recipe developed by Elissa Meadow. Solar Harvest, a premium, quick-casual restaurant that will offer a menu of natural, healthy cuisine items, will open in Los Angeles in spring 2005. For more restaurant information or for additional recipes, please visit www.solarharvestfood.com.

Turkey Kabobs

Prep: 20 minutes • Cook: 10 to 15 minutes

The tartness of the vinegar marinade for the vegetables complements the sweet citrus marinade for the meat. If you do not have access to an outdoor grill, I recommend using a stove-top grill pan or a broiler.

For the turkey and marinade:

> **1 pound boneless, skinless turkey breast**
>
> **1 orange, zested and juiced**
>
> **1 lemon, zested and juiced**
>
> **1 lime, zested and juiced**
>
> **2 teaspoons cumin**
>
> **2 teaspoons chili powder**
>
> **¼ cup olive oil**
>
> **Freshly ground black pepper, to taste**

For the vegetables and marinade:

> **1 red bell pepper, cut into 1 inch squares**
>
> **1 yellow bell pepper, cut into 1 inch squares**
>
> **1 large red onion, cut into wedges**
>
> **½ pound button mushrooms**
>
> **¼ cup olive oil**
>
> **3 tablespoons balsamic vinegar**
>
> **Freshly ground black pepper, to taste**

Preheat a barbecue grill.

To make the turkey: Cut the turkey breasts into 1-inch cubes. In a nonreactive bowl, whisk together all turkey marinade ingredients. Add the turkey and marinate, covered, in the refrigerator for 2 hours.

To make the vegetables: Whisk together the olive oil, balsamic vinegar, and pepper. Brush vegetables with the balsamic mixture.

Place vegetables and turkey on skewers, alternating vegetables as desired. Grill skewers for 10 to 15 minutes, rotating every few minutes, and brushing vegetables and turkey regularly with the appropriate marinade.

Makes 4 servings

Per serving: 360 calories, 22 g fat, 4 g saturated fat, 28 g protein, 14 g carbohydrates, 2 g dietary fiber, 75 mg cholesterol, 80 mg sodium

Recipe developed by Elissa Meadow.

Savory Stuffed Chicken Breasts

Prep: 5 minutes • Cook: 35 minutes

This couldn't be simpler or more appetizing. If you don't have wine or choose not to use it, substitute chicken broth. See Dining for One version on the opposite page.

> **Four 5-ounce skinless, boneless chicken breast halves**
>
> **1 package (4 ounces) light garlic- and herb-flavored cheese spread (such as Alouette)**
>
> **$\frac{1}{2}$ cup frozen chopped broccoli, thawed**
>
> **4 teaspoons dry white wine**
>
> **$\frac{1}{2}$ teaspoon salt**
>
> **$\frac{1}{4}$ teaspoon freshly ground black pepper**
>
> **1 bunch watercress, tough stems removed, rinsed and spun dry (about 4 loosely packed cups)**
>
> **$\frac{1}{4}$ cup chopped fresh tomato**
>
> **2 scallions, thinly sliced**

Preheat the oven to 375°F. Set out a rimmed baking sheet.

Place the chicken breasts on a cutting board. With a sharp knife, cut horizontally into the side of each breast to form a pocket, being careful not to slice all the way through. Open each up like a book.

In a small bowl, mix the cheese spread and broccoli. Spoon $\frac{1}{4}$ into the pocket in each chicken breast and smooth the top of the chicken over the filling.

Tear off four 14-inch-long pieces of heavy-duty foil. Fold each piece of foil crosswise, then open up.

In the center of each half, place a piece of chicken. Drizzle each with 1 teaspoon wine and sprinkle with salt and pepper.

Fold the other side of the foil over the chicken. Crimp the edges tightly to seal. Place the packets on the baking sheet. Bake until the chicken is no longer pink in the thickest part, about 25 minutes.

Meanwhile, divide the watercress among the dinner plates. Slide a chicken breast and any juices from the packet onto each plate and sprinkle each with some tomato and scallion. Serve.

Makes 4 servings

Per serving: 220 calories, 6 g fat, 3 g saturated fat, 36 g protein, 4 g carbohydrates, 0 g dietary fiber, 80 mg cholesterol, 520 mg sodium

Dining for One

One 5-ounce skinless, boneless chicken breast half

$2\frac{1}{2}$ tablespoons light garlic- and herb-flavored cheese spread (such as Alouette)

2 tablespoons thawed frozen chopped broccoli

1 teaspoon dry white wine

$\frac{1}{8}$ teaspoon salt

Pinch freshly ground black pepper

1 cup trimmed watercress

1 tablespoon each chopped fresh tomato and sliced scallion

Prepare as above and bake as directed.

Blueberry Bison (or Lean Beef) Burgers with Yam "Fries"

Prep: 25 minutes • Cook: 18 to 25 minutes

When you reveal the "secret" ingredient (blueberries) to your guests, everyone will be shocked. The blueberries make the burgers plump and juicy while also reducing the fat content by substituting meat with berries. If you have access to fresh-picked blueberries, use them. I make these burgers for summer barbecues with blueberries hand-picked by my nephew, and everyone asks for seconds.

Substituting cabbage leaves for buns and serving the burgers with Yam "Fries" provides a much healthier carbohydrate for the meal than either buns or fries made from regular potatoes, and the taste of the sweet yams compliments the tart blueberries well. If you are planning on entertaining, miniburger patties are great hors d'oeuvres for cocktail parties or Oscar parties. This recipe will make 12 to 16 miniburgers.

For the burgers:

½ cup blueberries

1 tablespoon balsamic vinegar

1 tablespoon mild Dijon mustard

1 teaspoon Worcestershire sauce

1 garlic clove, minced

Freshly ground black pepper, to taste

12 ounces ground bison meat or very lean ground beef

8 large outer leaves from a Napa cabbage

1 small red onion, sliced

1 red tomato, sliced

For the yams:

3 egg whites, lightly beaten

2 or 3 large Jewel Yams (can substitute sweet potatoes, but yams have a deeper orange color)

1 tablespoon sweet paprika

2 teaspoons cumin

Spicy Dijon mustard (optional)

To make the burgers: Preheat the broiler or barbecue grill.

In a food processor, puree the blueberries, vinegar, mustard, Worcestershire, garlic, and pepper. Combine pureed sauce with meat until blueberry puree is evenly distributed throughout meat.

Shape the mixture into 4 equally sized balls and then flatten the balls to create 4 patties.

Cook the patties either under the broiler or on the grill for 3 or 4 minutes per side, or until browned and no longer pink in the middle. Keep a close eye on the burgers since they cook more rapidly than all-meat burgers of the same size due to the amount of blueberries in the mixture. If burgers appear to be losing their moisture, remove from heat in order to preserve the juiciness.

While burgers are cooking, arrange 4 large Napa cabbage leaves on 4 plates, and top each leaf with a slice of onion and a slice of tomato.

When burgers are done, place patties on prepared cabbage leaves and top with desired mustards. Place the other cabbage leaves on top of the patties and serve with baked yam wedges (recipe below).

To make the yam fries: Preheat broiler and cover a baking sheet with foil.

Lightly beat the three egg whites with a fork or a whisk by hand.

Slice yams into thick wedges (6 to 10 per yam, depending on length of the yam. Longer yams should be halved before creating wedges.).

Brush fries with egg whites, creating a very light coating, avoiding getting too much egg on the skin side of the yams. Place yams, skin side down, on the baking sheet.

Sprinkle yam fries with paprika and cumin, and broil roughly 6 to 8 inches from heat source for 6 to 8 minutes, depending on preference for doneness. Longer cooking time allows fries to brown slightly more. Serve fries with mustard alongside blueberry burgers.

Makes 4 servings

Per serving: 370 calories, 14 g fat, 6 g saturated fat, 22 g protein, 41 g carbohydrates, 6 g dietary fiber, 60 mg cholesterol, 240 mg sodium

Blueberry Bison Burgers adapted by Elissa Meadow from Eating Well *magazine, winter 2004; Baked Yam Wedges developed by Elissa Meadow.*

Apple Betty

Prep: 2 minutes ● Cook: 3 minutes

This is a favorite of my clients. You can use the butter spray and the soda, or you can drizzle 1 teaspoon frozen apple juice concentrate over the crispbreads and another teaspoon over the apple. Either way, it's quick and easy.

> **2 GG Bran Crispbreads**
> **Butter-flavored spray**
> **Ground cinnamon**
> **1 medium Golden Delicious or Granny Smith apple, peeled,**
> **cored, and cut into thick slices**
> **2 tablespoons diet black cherry or cream soda (optional)**

In a small microwave-safe shallow dish, place the crispbreads. Mist with the butter-flavored spray and sprinkle with a pinch of cinnamon.

Arrange the apple slices on top and sprinkle with cinnamon. If desired, pour the soda over.

Cover with waxed paper and microwave on High until the apple is tender, about 2 minutes. Let stand a few minutes before serving.

Makes 1 serving

Per serving: 90 calories, 0 g fat, 0 g saturated fat, 2 g protein,
20 g carbohydrates, 5 g dietary fiber, 0 mg cholesterol, 0 mg sodium

Cinnamon-Pear Crumble

Prep: 10 minutes ● Bake: 1 hour, mostly unattended

This homey and comforting dessert is best made with very fragrant pears that feel a little soft when gently pressed. Serve with a dollop of nonfat vanilla yogurt, if you like. A Dining for One version follows.

> *For the pears:*
> **4 small firm-ripe pears (about 5 ounces each), peeled, cored, and**
> **cut in rough 1-inch chunks (about 4 cups)**
> **2 tablespoons thawed frozen apple juice concentrate**
> **¾ teaspoon ground cinnamon**

For the cinnamon crumble:
> ⅓ **cup old-fashioned oats**
> ¼ **teaspoon ground cinnamon**

To make the pears: Preheat the oven to 350°F. Set out four 4⅜ × 1³⁄₁₆-inch, 8-ounce aluminum "pot-pie pans" (found in the baking section of your grocery), or four 8-ounce custard cups, along with a baking sheet.

In a medium bowl, gently toss the pears, apple juice concentrate, and cinnamon. Divide evenly among the individual pans and place each on the baking sheet.

Bake until the pears are tender when pierced with a fork, 35 to 45 minutes (very ripe pears will cook more quickly). Transfer to a wire rack to cool. Leave the oven on.

To make the crumble: On a small baking sheet or baking pan, mix the oats and cinnamon. Bake, stirring once or twice, until very lightly toasted and crisp, about 10 minutes. Evenly spoon the crumble over the pears and serve warm or at room temperature.

Makes 4 servings

Per serving: 120 calories, 0.5 g fat, 0 g saturated fat, 2 g protein, 29 g carbohydrates, 5 g dietary fiber, 0 mg cholesterol, 0 mg sodium

Dining for One
> 1 **small firm-ripe pear (about 5 ounces), peeled, cored, and cut**
>   **in rough 1-inch chunks**
> 1½ **teaspoons thawed frozen apple juice concentrate**
> **Ground cinnamon**
> 1 **heaping tablespoon old-fashioned oats**

Preheat the oven to 350°F. In a 4⅜ × 1³⁄₁₆-inch, 8-ounce aluminum pot-pie pan or 8-ounce custard cup, mix the pear, apple juice concentrate, and ⅛ teaspoon cinnamon. Bake as directed above.

For the crumble, in a small nonstick skillet, stir the oats and a pinch of cinnamon. Cook over medium-low heat, stirring often, until just lightly toasted, about 3 minutes. Spoon over the pear and serve.

THE MAINTENANCE PHASE

By the time you're ready for the Maintenance Phase of the ABC Eating Plan, you should be within 2 to 3 pounds of your ideal weight. The C-list phase was created to help you come in for a safe landing as you approach your target.

The strategies and guidelines that have helped you lose weight apply even more on maintenance because your body is lighter and needs fewer calories than when you started. During maintenance, thinking historically, not just calorically, remains critical. As I've said throughout this book, the same people gain back the same weight on the same foods again and again. Just because you've lost weight and changed your size doesn't mean you've lost your vulnerability or changed your history with problem foods. *If, at any time during maintenance, you find that introducing a certain food(s) stimulates cravings and overconsumption, or you find that your appetite increases after you eat that food, eliminate it!*

I encourage you to read and reread the guidelines and protective strategies in the Tenth Commandment, Losing Weight Is Half the Job; Keeping It Off Is the Other Half. Complacency is the enemy of thin. You can eat the right foods, but if you don't practice the right behaviors, you'll just be another dieter who loses weight only to gain it back. To help protect you against this disappointment, I created the Maintenance New Scale as an early warning system. Weigh yourself daily or several times a week while on maintenance, and weigh your behavior and thinking weekly on the Maintenance New Scale. Truly, behavior predicts the direction your bathroom scale will be heading. That's why the Maintenance New Scale is such a unique and powerful tool in my work.

"How many calories can I add on maintenance?" is a question I'm frequently asked by clients before they start this phase of the eating plan. As most people approach their goal weight, they find that they're losing about a pound or two a week. Under these circumstances, you could normally add anywhere from 1,000 to 2,000 calories a week to your diet. Once again, the lower range applies to women, the higher range to men. If you're losing less than a pound a week, your body is probably telling you there's little room in your calorie budget for additions. At most, you may be looking to add an extra 500 calories a week. If your weight loss has stopped before or as you approach the goal and you still want to add new foods, you may do so one or two times a week. You may find that the day after you eat these foods, your weight is up. If it remains up for several days, return to the A-list eating until it drops to a lower number. Then you can add a new food or meal. It's like balancing a checkbook; if you overspend your calorie budget one day, you balance out the excess by returning to the A-list eating. Or, if you need more variety, you can switch to the B-list. The B-list foods may take several days longer to correct any weight gain. If the B-list doesn't do the job, stick with the A-list. Finally, if you're losing 2 pounds or more a week as you get nearer to the goal, you may be able to have between 2,000 (women) and 3,000 (men) calories a week, or a slightly higher amount. Once again, this is a simple balancing act. You add a new food or foods, and see if your weight goes up, down, or remains stable over the course of several days.

When you consider the best way to spend this calorie surplus, it's critical to think historically, not just calorically, especially if you come across a food you've chosen to Box Out or have abused in the past. I strongly urge you not to spend any of your maintenance calories on these foods. You don't need these foods for maintenance. What you need for maintenance is success.

Like you, my clients are unique people, and no two of them spend their calories exactly the same way. On maintenance, some add higher-caloric foods they feel they've been missing out on or would like to eat more often, such as sweet potatoes, olive oil, grains, alcohol, and bananas. Others spend their calories on desserts, provided they're desserts that they have no history of abusing. Some of you may find that you don't miss anything and decide to stay with the menus and foods from the first two phases of the diet.

Some General Food Considerations on Maintenance

During this phase of the eating plan, white and green still equal lean. A basic cornerstone of your diet should still be the low-fat white protein and green and white vegetables you started with on the 10-Day TurboCharge Diet. These will always be the best choices for maintaining a healthy weight, guarding control, and giving structure to your eating. To help you simplify your food and meal decisions on maintenance, I've provided you with guidelines for many popular foods you may have questions about or are thinking of adding to your diet.

On maintenance, for example, you can add 1 or 2 tablespoons of the "good fats" in vegetable oil, such as olive or canola, a day. A large number of my clients typically use about 1 tablespoon of oil while losing weight. For many of them, this would be a second or third tablespoon a day. Many find they can prepare their vegetables with oil and not gain weight. On the other hand, some of my clients find that steaming their vegetables is a better use of their calorie budget and forgoing oil leaves them room to spend on other foods. If you strongly prefer butter to oil, you can use one pat of butter a day. For health purposes, I infinitely prefer you use one of the butter substitutes I recommend, a low-fat yogurt/butter mix, or a margarine such as Smart Balance, which contains no hydrogenated fat and tastes similar to butter.

If you like bagels, and you're confident that eating them won't lead you back into abusing breads or breadbaskets, you can have one or two a week on maintenance, although I suggest that you "Box Them In" to weekends. I recommend weekends because most bagels, even the whole-wheat variety, are high in calories and not a food you want to get used to eating too often. You may also want to try the new "light bagels" now available, which may have substantially fewer calories than regular bagels. Men can have a maximum of two bagels a week; women can have one. Of course, if you want to save even more calories, have an English muffin or a bialy.

On the question of bread, it's always best to continue using the GG Scandinavian Bran Crispbread or similar bran cracker. However, if you choose bread, I still want you using the light bread choices I recommend on the B-List phase of the eating plan. If a light bread isn't available, you can have two slices of regular calorie bread (80 to 100 calories a slice) one or two times a week.

If you're going to a sporting event or picnic, it's always best to eat something beforehand. However, I don't mind if you have one hamburger or hot dog with a bun or half a bun (unless you've Boxed Out bread). But you should count this as one of your weekly gourmet meals. And you should always avoid chips, fries, buttered popcorn, and other snack foods that are often widely available at sporting events and picnics. If you're bent on snacking, bring a low-calorie, healthy option such as an apple, four or five bran crackers, two or three wedges of fat-free or low-fat cheese, or one of the "light" popcorns I recommend.

Avoid deep-fried foods such as french fries and onion rings—staples of the modern American diet—altogether or eat them infrequently (for both caloric and health reasons). If you really want fries, there are some brands of baked fries and fat-free french fries available in the freezer section of many major supermarket chains. For an even healthier alternative, try my fried zucchini chips (page 219). If you prefer baked or boiled potatoes, you can have from one to seven medium-size baked or boiled potatoes a week, but no more than one a day on maintenance.

As you may already know from the B-list foods guidelines, I'm no great fan of breakfast cereals since people tend to take two or three times the recommended serving size. This is especially the case when people are on maintenance and no longer concerned with the number of pounds they lose each week. Steer clear of cereals that contain dried fruit, which may appear to be healthy, but do little except add on calories. Remember the "Rule of Five." If a cereal has more than 5 grams of sugar and less than 5 grams of dietary fiber per serving, you'll know immediately it's not a nutritious choice. Men can have a single, measured serving to a serving and a half of cereal every day; women may have a single serving of cereal one to five times a week.

And as far as desserts are concerned, I suggest that you continue to follow the light gourmet dessert recipes, or use a low-calorie, store-bought dessert that comes in a fixed amount, such as the Weight Watchers Smart Ones New York Style Cheesecake or Patisserie de France Giurees. If you want higher-calorie desserts, it's best to eat them at a restaurant, where you only get individual servings. If sugar is a major issue for you, I urge that dessert consist only of fruit, a cappuccino with whipped cream, or one of my special dessert recipes you feel comfortable with. Woman can have one higher-calorie dessert a week, and men can have two. Just remember that frequent consumption of products with added cane sugar or fructose may lead to increased appetite and cravings.

While the foods are important from a caloric point of view, how often you eat them may be even *more* important from a control point

(continued on page 278)

Phase C: Maintenance Food Guidelines

Avoid all foods you have a history of abusing and that you have Boxed Out. Remember to limit the frequency and quantity of foods you have Boxed In—you have lost weight, not your vulnerability to these foods.

Food	Women	Men
Alcohol (excluding drinks that include fruit juice, tonic water, or regular soda)	Occasional use; no more than 1 time a day suggested maximum	Occasional use; no more than 2 times a day suggested maximum
Bagels (suggest a bialy or English muffin)	For occasional use (once a week, preferably on weekends) or avoid	For occasional use (twice a week, preferably on weekends) or avoid
Breakfast cereal (including oatmeal)	A single, measured serving of a high-fiber cereal that contains no added sugar (must be less than 5g of sugar and more than 5g of fiber), 1–5 times a week	Same instruction as for women, but every day
Butter and margarine	Avoid butter, or use no more than 1 pat. Avoid margarines with hydrogenated or partially hydrogenated oil. If margarine is used in lieu of oil, limit to 1–2 times a day	Same instructions as for women, but 3–4 times a day
Candy	To be used infrequently or on special occasions; best to choose Gayle's Chocolate Truffles, a Tootsie Pop, or Dream Bar	Same instructions as for women
Desserts	For occasional use or avoid. If you want to have desserts more frequently, choose something from the phase A or B menu, or a Weight Watchers dessert	For occasional use or avoid. Same instruction as for women

Food	Women	Men
French fries	Avoid or for occasional use only	Avoid or for occasional use only
Fruits (except grapes, cherries, or cut-up fruit)	2–3 a day	3–4 a day
Fruit juice (in lieu of a serving of fruit)	4–6 ounces a day	6–8 ounces a day
Full-calorie gourmet meals	1–2 a week	3–4 a week
Olive oil or similar vegetable oil	1–2 Tbsp a day	2–3 Tbsp a day
Pasta (counts as a full-calorie gourmet meal)	Avoid pasta made with Alfredo sauce, cheese, or oil; maximum of 4 oz once a week, or a 2-oz appetizer twice a week	Avoid pasta made with Alfredo sauce, cheese, or oil; maximum of 5 oz once a week, or a 2- to 3-oz appetizer twice a week
Pizza (counts as a gourmet meal)	Only choose a cheese or vegetable topping; 1 slice a week	Only choose a cheese or vegetable topping; 2 slices a week
Potato or grains	1 medium potato (preferably boiled and sweet) or ½ cup of grains, 1–3 times a week	1 medium potato or ¾ cup of grains, 2–7 times a week
Salad dressings	Prepare with 1 Tbsp of olive oil	Prepare with 1–2 Tbsp of olive oil
Sandwiches	Occasional use or prepare with 2 slices of light bread or GG Crispbreads	Occasional use or prepare with 2 slices of light bread or GG Crispbreads
Snack foods or desserts from the list of recommended foods (page 279)	Up to 3 times a day	Maximum of 4 times a day
Tomato sauce (without oil)	Use as needed	Use as needed

of view. If you eat a certain food over and over again, such as pasta or bread, you may come to expect it regularly, or it may become part of your daily menu. Be aware of this reality of eating behavior. If adding a certain food to your diet might cause you to eat too much, avoid that food or Box It In to weekends, holidays, and special events.

On the maintenance phase, women can typically have two gourmet meals a week, and men are allowed three or four. These meals would include foods served with sauce or gravy. So, if you plan on dining out, you don't have to make any special preparations (except never to go hungry). However, if you have a meal with sauce or gravy at home, either choose an alternative from the recipe list or count it as one of your gourmet entrées.

After you eat some of the higher-calorie meals and foods on maintenance, you might find that your weight jumps 2 or 3 pounds. Don't be alarmed. Part of this may be water retention from salt, which will dissipate itself. For many people, it's normal to gain a few pounds, especially after an elaborate meal at a nice restaurant or special event. If this happens to you, *simply return to the A-list or B-list foods Monday through Friday;* the weight will come off, and you can return to higher-calorie choices on weekends. By "higher-calorie choices," I mean foods prepared with sauces, a higher-fat meat dish, higher-carbohydrate foods such as pasta or lasagna, or a plate of shrimp tempura. Another gourmet choice could be the *taster menu*—hopefully minus the breadbasket and dessert—at your favorite gourmet restaurant.

Continue to think in terms of your calorie budget if you decide to have alcohol. Remember, just one drink a day can cost you around 3,000 calories a month. Try to avoid alcoholic fruit drinks and drinks made with tonic and regular soda, since they often contain double the amount of calories as drinks made with water or club soda. Women can have one drink a day; men can have two.

As you enjoy the nearly limitless variety of foods and gourmet meals on this eating plan, you should be constantly reminded that weight control doesn't mean giving up the pleasure of great food. Living thin is not about magic. Rather, it's about being smart and selective and using your calorie budget wisely, so you can have the greatest foods in the world, while also enjoying a lifetime of being in control of your eating . . . and being trim.

Bon appétit!

Snacks and Desserts for Phase C

Some of these choices tend to be higher in calories or carbohydrates than those on the other two phases of the plan. These are for occasional use or at special events.

Snacks and Desserts

Chef Miriam's Angel Cake
  See recipe, page 290.

Weight Watchers Smart Ones New York Style Cheesecake (150 calories each)

Lay's Original Fat-Free Potato Chips (individual bags have 75 calories)

Restaurant Desserts

No more than once a week (unless your dessert is fruit or a scoop of sorbet without cookies)

Cheese Crepes with Blueberry Sauce
  See recipe, page 288.

Chef Miriam's Raspberry Soufflé
  See recipe, page 291.

Dream Bar (90-calorie chocolate bar)

The Dessert Dilemma: Keeping the Tradition without the Trouble

For some people, dessert is one of the more pleasurable parts of the dining experience. Whether you're eating at home with your family or enjoying a fine meal at your favorite restaurant, more often than not, dessert will be on the menu. Some of you may not consider a special meal complete unless it culminates with a piece of cake, a few scoops of ice cream, or a cream-filled éclair.

This universal tradition of serving desserts is the Achilles' heel of many dieters and weight clients. They want to be included in all the merriment surrounding celebrations and special meals and may feel deprived if they don't partake in dessert. Aside from the excessive calories, carbohydrates, and saturated fat in many popular desserts, the other problem is that people tend to abuse and overeat dessert foods or compulsively nibble on the leftovers, especially while they're cleaning up after a dinner party or event at their home.

By now, you might be thinking to yourself, "How do I keep the tradition I love without all the trouble?" Perhaps the safest move is to serve festive, fruit-based desserts, such as our cinnamon baked apple, or yogurt parfait made with Total Yogurt, fruit, and Walden Farms Calorie-Free Chocolate Syrup. Or, you may opt for a piece of my Strawberry Shortcake (page 85). These desserts are low in calories, delicious, pleasing to the eye, seldom abused—and people love them.

If you don't have the time or inclination to prepare dessert, you can select any one of the 20 or so ready-made choices from the shopping list (page 294). I'm especially fond of the Patisserie de France Orange and Lemon Giurees (orange and lemon skins filled with sorbet that weigh in at 89 and 65 calories respectively). Many of my clients enjoy the Giurees and often serve them to rave reviews at family dinners and special events.

If you decide to serve a baked dessert but are concerned about abusing it or adding excess calories to your diet, there a couple of things you might want to consider beforehand.

- It's better to buy than to bake. Try to avoid purchasing desserts that need to be prepared, such as cakes, brownies, and cookies. However, if you need or choose to bake, try Chef Miriam's Angel Cake or one of our other light desserts. They are loved, but seldom abused.
- Beware the baker's oven. If you go to a bakery to pick up a dessert, try to avoid doing so late in the day when your blood sugar might be

low or you might be hungry and tempted to overbuy.

- Only buy baked goods that come in individual servings (such as tarts, cupcakes, or brownies). If you're having company, buy only what you need for each guest, and if baked goods are an issue for you, serve yourself something you don't have a history of abusing. Single servings will keep you from picking at left-overs. If cookies are your issue, you should avoid them entirely. They are the most frequently abused baked goods along with all bite-size baked goods such as mini-pastries. You should only buy the *exact* amount you need for your guests so there are no extras. You can also ask your local ice cream store or bakery to prepare a frozen low-fat cake or yo-gurt pie without the crust. For birthday parties, many of my clients who are trying to avoid cakes buy a large cake they don't like or purchase smaller, individually packaged cakes (or cupcakes) for each of their guests.
- Freezing won't protect you; it'll only delay the inevitable. If you have a history of abusing baked goods, don't assume that putting them in deep storage will protect you. It'll only delay trouble.

If you're trying to avoid dessert, and you attend a dinner party, wed-ding, or other special event, always ask your waiter not to bring you any dessert as he clears away your entrée. Even if you're resolved not to have dessert, you're likely to nibble or pick at something if it's put in front of you. If you feel compelled or obligated to have a dessert, ask for fresh fruit, a single scoop of sorbet (specify without cookies), or cup of cappuccino with light whipped cream.

At a restaurant, try to avoid reading the dessert menu altogether (unless it's your birthday or other unique occa-sion). If you're concerned about avoiding sweets, the safest dessert at a restaurant is a food you're unlikely to see every day or one that's difficult to come by, such as a chocolate or vanilla mousse or crème brulee. A safe way to sample but avoid excess calories is to order one dessert for the table and have everyone share. Perhaps the best strategy is simply to wait and have one of our light desserts at home.

Whatever the occasion, using a little strategy will keep you from having to wear what you eat the next day. Now, the next time you blow out the candles on your birthday, you won't have to wish to be thin.

Authentic Huevos Rancheros with Sauce and Guacamole

Prep: 30 minutes • Cook: 35 minutes

Huevos Rancheros adds excitement to any brunch or breakfast. Use corn tortillas made from pure cornmeal to reduce the use of processed foods and to ensure the crispiness of the tortillas. I developed the guacamole recipe through many taste trials, and its easy preparation makes it a wonderful addition to lunch or dinner either to accompany fajitas or to serve with hors d'oeuvres. To make this a lower-carb meal, you can either use less of the bean mixture or forego the tortillas all together.

For the ranchero sauce:

> **2 teaspoons olive oil**
>
> **1 small onion, chopped**
>
> **1 jalapeño chile, chopped (if desire less heat, remove seeds and ribs)**
>
> **1 garlic clove, minced**
>
> **1 can (14.5 ounces) crushed tomatoes**

For the guacamole:

> **2 ripe avocados**
>
> **¼ cup minced onion**
>
> **1 jalapeño chile, chopped (if desire less heat, remove seeds and ribs)**
>
> **2 plum tomatoes, seeded and diced**
>
> **¼ teaspoon cayenne**
>
> **1 teaspoon chile powder**
>
> **Juice of 2 limes**
>
> **2 tablespoons cilantro, chopped, or to taste**
>
> **Tabasco sauce, to taste**

For the huevos:

> **4 corn tortillas (if desired)**
>
> **1 can (16 ounces) black beans with their liquid**
>
> **Cooking spray**
>
> **8 eggs**
>
> **½ cup shredded chipotle or Monterey Jack cheese**
>
> **2 tablespoons chopped cilantro**
>
> **Ranchero Sauce (see recipe opposite)**
>
> **Guacamole (see recipe opposite)**

To make the ranchero sauce: Heat the oil in a medium saucepan. Add the onions and cook until just barely translucent. Stir in the jalapeño and garlic. Sauté for 1 or 2 more minutes, until the jalapeño releases its scent. Add the tomatoes and cook until heated through.

Keep the sauce warm over low heat until ready to serve with the Huevos Rancheros.

To make the guacamole: Quarter the avocados and remove the skin, reserving the pits. Using an avocado masher or the back of a fork, mash avocados until only a few lumps remain. Add the onion, jalapeño, and diced tomatoes and combine until well mixed with the mashed avocados. Add cayenne, chile powder, and lime juice. Combine well.

Mix in the cilantro and Tabasco to taste, and salt, if desired.

Place pits back in bowl to preserve color. Serve with Huevos Rancheros or Chicken or Steak Fajitas (page 264).

To make the huevos: Preheat the oven to 450°F.

Place corn tortillas on a baking sheet and bake until slightly crisp, 4 to 7 minutes. When tortillas are done, place them on 4 plates.

Place beans in a small saucepan and heat until heated through. Do not bring liquid to a boil. When beans are heated, leave over low heat until ready to serve.

Heat a nonstick pan over high heat and spray with a light layer of cooking spray. Fry the eggs, two at a time, until whites are firm and yolks are slightly loose, 1 to 2 minutes. If desired, flip eggs for 30 seconds to cook more. Transfer eggs to prepared tortilla plates when finished.

Spoon ¼ to ½ cup of heated beans over eggs, followed by cheese and cilantro. Spoon generous amounts of the heated rancheros sauce over the top. Spoon guacamole in a ball on top and serve with extra bowls of ranchero sauce and guacamole.

Makes 4 servings

Per serving: 550 calories, 32 g fat, 8 g saturated fat, 26 g protein, 50 g carbohydrates, 16 g dietary fiber, 435 mg cholesterol, 650 mg sodium

Huevos, sauce, and guacamole recipes developed by Elissa Meadow. Solar Harvest, a premium, quick-casual restaurant that will offer a menu of natural, healthy cuisine items, will open in Los Angeles in spring 2005. For more restaurant information or for additional recipes, please visit www.solarharvestfood.com.

Waffles Supreme with Ricotta and Raspberry Sauce

Prep: 4 minutes • Cook: 10 minutes

This is terrific for Sunday brunch. If Van's waffles aren't available, choose another waffle with about 100 calories each. The sauce can be made a day or so ahead and reheated in the microwave just before serving.

1¼ cups frozen unsweetened raspberries

1 tablespoon water

2 teaspoons Splenda

4 Van's waffles

¼ cup fat-free ricotta cheese

Ground cinnamon

In a medium microwave-safe bowl, mix the raspberries, water, and Splenda. Cover with vented plastic wrap and microwave on High for 1 minute. Stir. Microwave for 1 minute longer, until the berries are hot and begin to release juices. Cover to keep warm.

To serve, toast the waffles and spread each with 1 tablespoon ricotta. Sprinkle with a little cinnamon and top each with about 2 tablespoons sauce. Serve right away.

Makes 4 servings (⅔ cup sauce)

Per serving: 140 calories, 2.5 g fat, 0 g saturated fat, 4 g protein, 21 g carbohydrates, 4 g dietary fiber, 5 mg cholesterol, 220 mg sodium

The Diet Doctor's 25 Favorite Foods

Have you ever wondered what a diet doctor eats and keeps in his own home? These are the 25 foods that I have found work best for great taste, weight control, and great health.

1. Fage Total 2% Greek Yogurt
2. Chicken: My personal favorites are Tyson Italian-Style Tasty Selections Boneless and Skinless Chicken Breasts, Perdue Fit 'N Easy Skinless and Boneless Chicken Breasts, and Perdue Low-Fat Breaded Italian-Style Chicken Cutlets
3. GG Scandinavian Bran Crisp-breads and Bran-a-Crisp crackers
4. Envelopes of water-packed tuna, especially chunk light and white meat Albacore
5. Seafood, especially shrimp, lobster, crab, and white meat fishes
6. Van's Multigrain Belgian Waffles
7. Green and white vegetables, not including potato and avocado (made without butter or oil)
8. Eggs, especially egg whites and egg substitutes
9. Alba Protein Shakes (made with either water or fat-free milk)
10. Oscar Mayer Fat-Free Hot Dogs and Hebrew National 97% Fat-Free Hot Dogs
11. I Can't Believe It's Not Butter spray
12. Gayle's Chocolate Truffles (only for company)
13. Diet soda, especially Jeff's Diet Chocolate Soda and Stewart's Diet Orange Soda
14. Butterball Thin 'N Crispy Turkey Bacon
15. Laughing Cow Light Cheese
16. Chocolate Mousse Pops: Yoplait Chocolate Mousse Pop, Skinny Cow Fat-Free Fudge Bar, Klondike Carb-Smart Fudge and Ice Cream Bar (or ice cream sandwich)
17. Walden Farms Calorie-Free Chocolate Dip or Syrup
18. Patisserie de France Giurees (orange or lemon skins filled with delicious sorbet for about 90 and 60 calories respectively)
19. Walden Farms Thick 'N Spicy Barbecue Sauce and Walden Farms Salad Dressings (especially balsamic)
20. Light cold cuts, especially Hebrew National Lean Salami, Hillshire Farms Light Pastrami, Oscar Mayer Fat-Free Bologna, Healthy Choice Ham, Hormel Turkey Pepperoni, and Ives Veggie Pepperoni
21. Morningstar Tomato & Basil Pizza Burgers
22. Celestial Seasonings Chai Tea (with cinnamon)
23. Swiss Miss Diet Hot Chocolate (25 calories)
24. Kellogg's All-Bran with Extra Fiber
25. Imagine Free-Range Chicken Broth

Roasted Organic Turkey Breast

Prep: 20 minutes ● Cook: 2½ to 4½ hours

I've adapted this recipe for my mother's famous turkey breast to reduce the processed sugars used while still maintaining the flavor. Using pure fruit jam eliminates the refined sugars, and though making the sauce may seem labor-intensive, the added flavor is well worth it. I've also substituted olive oil for butter to eliminate the dairy component for those who are lactose-intolerant. However, you may substitute a more neutral oil, such as canola or grapeseed, if you want a more subtle flavor. This turkey-breast meat is great for homemade sandwiches and panini or to top a fresh salad.

1 can crushed tomatoes (28 ounces)

1 cup water

1 cup white vinegar

¼ cup pure-fruit apricot jam (fruit and juices only, such as
 Sorrel Ridge)

Juice of 2 oranges

Juice of 2 limes

2 tablespoons Dijon mustard

1 tablespoon Worcestershire sauce

2 teaspoons onion powder

1 teaspoon chili powder

1 clove garlic, minced

½ teaspoon cayenne pepper

1 can beer (12 ounces)

4 tablespoons olive oil

1 medium (4 to 6 pounds) organic turkey breast, bone in

Chopped fresh herbs for seasoning (choice of any mix of parsley,
 thyme, rosemary, basil, oregano)

Preheat oven to 325°F.

In a medium saucepan, combine the tomatoes, water, vinegar, apricot jam, orange and lime juices, mustard, Worcestershire sauce, onion powder, chili powder, garlic, and cayenne pepper. Simmer over low heat for 30 minutes.

Add the beer and olive oil and simmer for another 15 to 20 minutes.

Season the turkey breast with the fresh herbs, then baste with the sauce.

Place turkey in oven and baste every 15 minutes, until turkey is done (1½ to 2 hours). Test for doneness by sticking a fork in the turkey. If juices are clear, remove turkey from oven.

Slice turkey breast and serve as desired.

Makes 8 servings

Per serving: 480 calories, 19 g fat, 4 g saturated fat, 33 g protein, 40 g carbohydrates, 2 g dietary fiber, 90 mg cholesterol, 490 mg sodium

Recipe developed by Elissa Meadow. Solar Harvest, a premium, quick-casual restaurant that will offer a menu of natural, healthy cuisine items, will open in Los Angeles in spring 2005. For more restaurant information or for additional recipes, please visit www.solarharvestfood.com.

Cheese Crepes with Blueberry Sauce

Prep: 15 minutes ● Cook: 25 minutes

All of the elements of this delectable dessert can be prepared in advance, wrapped, and refrigerated. Only the sauce should be warm—simply reheat it in the microwave.

For the crepes:

½ cup skim milk

2 large egg whites

¼ cup plus 1 tablespoon whole grain pastry flour

¼ teaspoon ground cinnamon

⅛ teaspoon salt

For the cheese filling:

4 ounces (½ cup) fat-free cream cheese

½ cup fat-free ricotta cheese

1 teaspoon grated lemon zest

½ teaspoon Splenda

For the blueberry sauce:

1½ cups fresh or frozen blueberries

3 tablespoons light sugar-free boysenberry, strawberry, or raspberry preserves

1 tablespoon water

To prepare the crepe batter: In a blender, place the skim milk, egg whites, flour, cinnamon, and salt. Whirl at high speed until smooth. Let stand while making the filling and sauce.

To make the filling: In a small bowl, mash the cream cheese, ricotta, lemon zest, and Splenda with the back of a fork until well blended.

To make the sauce: In a small saucepan, stir the blueberries, preserves, and water. Cook over medium heat, stirring often, until the berries have softened and the sauce boils, 5 to 8 minutes. (Fresh berries will cook faster than frozen.) Cover and set aside to keep warm.

To make the crepes: Coat a small nonstick skillet (7 inches across the top) with cooking spray. Heat over medium heat for 1 minute. Reduce the heat to medium-low.

Stir the batter and spoon 2 measuring tablespoons into the pan, swirling to coat the bottom evenly. Cook until the edges are golden brown, about 1½ minutes. Carefully loosen the edges with a nylon spatula; turn and cook about 30 seconds longer. Slide onto a plate. Repeat, making 8 crepes, spraying the pan once more, if necessary.

To serve, spoon 2 tablespoons filling into the center of each crepe and roll up. Serve 2 crepes per person, topped with ¼ cup sauce each.

Makes 4 servings (8 crepes, ½ cup filling, 1 cup sauce)

Per serving: 150 calories, 1 g fat, 0 g saturated fat, 11 g protein, 25g carbohydrates, 3 g dietary fiber, 10 mg cholesterol, 300 mg sodium

Angel Cakes

Prep: 5 minutes ● Cook: 30 minutes

Serve each cake with a few slices of strawberry and fresh peaches or nectarines. For tips on using egg whites, see the Raspberry Soufflé recipe on the opposite page.

> **4 large egg whites, at room temperature**
> **⅛ teaspoon cream of tartar**
> **⅛ teaspoon salt**
> **⅓ cup Splenda**
> **½ teaspoon vanilla extract**
> **¼ teaspoon almond extract**
> **⅔ cup whole grain pastry flour**

Preheat the oven to 325°F. Coat four 4⅜- × 1³⁄₁₆-inch, 8-ounce aluminum "pot-pie pans" (found in the baking section of your grocery) with cooking spray. Place on a baking sheet.

With an electric mixer at medium speed, beat the egg whites, cream of tartar, and salt until frothy. Increase the speed to high and gradually beat in the Splenda. Continue beating until glossy stiff peaks form when the beater is lifted. Beat in the extracts to blend. Sift about half the flour over the beaten whites. With a large rubber spatula, fold in the flour until blended. Repeat with the remaining flour. With a small rubber spatula, divide the batter evenly among the prepared pans. Gently smooth the tops.

Bake until firm, very lightly browned, and a toothpick inserted in the center comes out clean, about 20 minutes. Transfer to wire racks to cool completely. Turn out of the pans to serve.

Makes 4 servings

Per serving: 100 calories, 0 g fat, 0 g saturated fat, 6 g protein, 18 g carbohydrates, 3 g dietary fiber, 0 mg cholesterol, 130 mg sodium

Raspberry Soufflé

Prep: 8 minutes • Cook: 35 minutes

Wow, this is a showstopper—just don't tell anyone how easy it is. This gorgeous dessert is perfect for a small dinner party or family event. Serve with tiny cups of espresso.

Note: To ensure that egg whites beat properly, they must be free of any egg yolk. Plus, the mixer bowl needs to be very clean. Wipe the bowl and beaters with a paper towel lightly moistened with white vinegar before using.

> ¾ cup fresh raspberries
>
> 3 tablespoons light sugar-free raspberry preserves
>
> 4 large egg whites, at room temperature (see note)
>
> ⅛ teaspoon cream of tartar
>
> Pinch salt
>
> ¼ cup Splenda

Preheat the oven to 400°F. Coat six 5- or 6-ounce soufflé dishes or oven-proof ramekins with cooking spray and place on a rimmed baking sheet.

In a large bowl, mash the raspberries and preserves to a fairly smooth puree (a little texture is good) with a fork or wire whisk.

With an electric mixer at medium speed, beat the egg whites, cream of tartar, and salt until frothy. Increase the speed to high and gradually beat in the Splenda. Continue beating until glossy stiff peaks form.

With a large rubber spatula, fold the beaten whites into the raspberry puree until no white streaks remain. With a smaller spatula, evenly spoon the mixture into the prepared dishes (they will be very full). Run your finger through the batter once in a circular pattern to even it out.

Bake until golden brown, firm to the touch and well risen, 10 to 12 minutes. Remove from the oven. With a metal spatula, transfer each dish to a small plate and serve at once.

Makes 6 servings

Per serving: 30 calories, 0 g fat, 0 g saturated fat, 3 g protein, 5 g carbohydrates, 0 g dietary fiber, 0 mg cholesterol, 35 mg sodium

Alcohol: Strategies to Keep the Calories from Adding Up

Dieters are no different than most people, and some may like to have a drink every now and then. It often helps them to relax and unwind, especially after a tough day at work. However, if you're concerned about your weight, watching your alcohol intake can be important. I remind my clients who like to have a drink every day that it could cost them as many as 3,500 calories a month—that's an extra 10 pounds a year. While it may not be my favorite use of calories, a limited amount of alcohol doesn't have to impair your control or blow your calorie budget, provided you follow a few guidelines.

When choosing a drink, try picking one that's low in calories. If, for example, you're accustomed to having one beer a night with dinner, simply switching from regular to light beer may save you upward of 50 to 60 calories. Always avoid tonic and juice drinks (especially margaritas unless you count them as "dessert in a glass"). Some of my savviest calorie-counting clients replace one of their snacks or minimeals with a glass of alcohol each day to save calories. From a nutritional and appetite-control point of view, this is probably not the best way to use your calorie budget.

Throughout this book, we have looked at foods not just in terms of the number of calories they contain but in the way they affect your behavior. Alcohol is an ideal case for this phenomenon. Some of my clients tell me that alcohol saves them from nibbling on a breadbasket or munching on hors d'oeuvres. Others, especially women, tell me that if they drink on an empty stomach, they're more likely to snack uncontrollably, make poor food decisions, or order a high-calorie dessert. Once again, thinking historically, not just calorically, will give you the answer. Look at your own history with alcohol, and see which of these behaviors, if any, applies directly to you.

A further issue with alcohol is that it lowers your inhibitions and may make some of you more likely to eat dessert or select foods you have chosen to "Box Out" or have a history of abusing. *I've found that this is more apt to occur if you drink on an empty stomach or drink before your meal.* So if alcohol has this effect on you, particularly if you're at a restaurant or social situation, save your drink for the meal. If, on the other hand, you feel you must have a drink when you first arrive at a social event or party, perhaps to reduce any social anxiety, eat something beforehand, so you're not consuming alcohol on an empty stomach.

Since the amount we drink is often tied to how long we spend talking or socializing, always order two drinks—one alcoholic, the other not—when you place a drink order. This way you can alternate sips of the alcoholic and nonalcoholic drinks. Also, try to avoid having two alcoholic drinks in a row because people who have one drink after another will consume a lot more during the course of an evening. Having multiple drinks, particularly on an empty stomach, can wreak havoc with your blood-sugar levels. This effect can stimulate your appetite by increasing levels of the hunger hormone insulin or impair your ability to refrain from breadbaskets or hors d'oeuvres or even order a proper meal. You may also find that drinking increases the likelihood of ordering a dessert.

Another insider tip to limit your alcohol intake is to *drink what you don't like*. I've observed that people who order what they like "drink" instead of sip and usually consume a lot more. So if you're drinking just to relax or to be more social, you're likely to consume

less if it's something you don't love. For example, some of my male clients who take in too many calories from alcohol have found that switching from vodka to bourbon or white wine causes them to consume fewer drinks. My female clients seem to do better with red than white wine or switching from wine to scotch or rum.

If you're drinking harder liquor, mix it with a beverage containing few or no calories. Scotch and club soda or vodka and club soda will make the drink last longer and slow the impact of the alcohol. Also, avoid mixing your alcohol with fruit juice, tonic, or nondiet soda, which can add anywhere from 100 to 150 calories to your drink.

Finally, drinking at dinner or during the evening may interfere with your sleep cycle and cause you to get up during the night. So if you're someone who likes to eat during the night, you need to be careful. This is especially the case with sugar abusers who find that alcohol causes them to crave sweets.

No matter what, when, or where you choose to drink, using good strategy can keep a little imbibing from turning into an evening you may soon want to forget.

Taste Is King Awards: The 110 Best Light Foods on the Market

These are the very best light foods on the market that give great taste without great calories. Once you try them, you'll realize why I say, "It's not about deprivation but substitution."

1 Fage Total Yogurt

2 Gayle's Miracles Perfect Chocolate Truffles

3 Fruit H_2O Frozen Ices

4 Jeff's Diet Chocolate Soda

5 Dannon Light 'n Fit Carb Control Vanilla Cream Yogurt

6 Walden Farms Calorie-Free Dips (especially Chocolate and Marshmallow)

7 Perdue Low-Fat Breaded Italian Style Chicken Cutlets

8 Perdue Low-Fat Homestyle Chicken Cutlets

9 Alba Fit n' Frosty Shakes

10 Walden Farms Calorie-Free Honey Dijon Dressing

11 Van's 7-Grain Belgian Waffles

12 Butterball Thin & Crispy Turkey Bacon

13 Walden Farms Calorie-Free Thick N Spicy BBQ Sauce

14 Tyson Italian Style Tasty Selections Boneless & Skinless Chicken Breasts

15 Country Cottage Sugar-Free Maple Syrup

16 Celentano Lite Eggplant Rollatini

17 Oscar Mayer Fat-Free Bologna

18 The Skinny Cow Fat-Free Fudge Bar

19 Thomas Light English Muffins

20 Lifesavers Sugar-Free Flavor Pops

21 Jell-O Sugar-Free Pops

22 Fat-Free Reddi-wip

23 Swiss Miss Diet Hot Chocolate or Carnation Hot Chocolate Light

24 Oscar Mayer Fat-Free All Beef Frankfurters

25 Hormel Turkey Pepperoni

26 Hebrew National Lean Salami

27 Hebrew National 97% Fat-Free Franks

28 Butterball Fat-Free Turkey Franks

29 Amy's Organic Shepherd's Pie

30 Amy's Veggie Meatloaf

31 Beefsteak Rye Bread Soft Light

32 Lipton Diet Peach Ice Tea

33 Dr. Praeger's Veggie Burgers

34 Boca Breakfast Links

35 Morningstar Tomato & Basil Pizza Burgers

36 Tasters Choice Instant Flavored Coffees

37 Ocean Beauty Salmon Burgers

38 Walden Farms Balsamic Vinaigrette

39 Gardenburger Portobello Mushroom & Original Flavor

40 Knight's Light Popcorn

41 President's Fat-Free Feta Cheese

42 Hillshire Farms Light 'n Lean Cold Cuts (especially bologna, pastrami, and corned beef)

43 Instafiber Tea Drink

44 Kellogg's All-Bran with Extra Fiber

45 Walden Farms Calorie-Free Salad Dressings (in individual packets)

46 Joseph's Sugar-Free Cookies

47 Smart Beat Soy Cheese

48 Calabro Brothers Fat-Free Ricotta and Mozzarella

49 Smuckers Light Sugar-Free Preserves

50 Cowboy Caviar's Veggie Tomato dips

51 Norseland Lite Cheese

52 Promise Ultra Light Margarine

53 Hellman's Just 2 Good Mayonnaise

54 Polly-O Reduced-Fat Shredded Mozzarella

55 V-8 Spicy Hot and Low Sodium Veggie Juice

56 D'Artagnan Chicken Sausages

57 Pam Olive Oil Spray

58 Trader Joe's Sweet Italian Sausage

59 Van de Kamp's Crisp & Healthy Fish Sticks

60 Gorton's Cajun Blackened Grilled Fish Fillets

61 Aunt Jemima Low-Fat Pancakes

62 Trader Joe's Tuna Burgers or Salmon Patties

63 Weight Watchers Smart Ones Pops Chocolate Mousse and Orange Vanilla Treat

64 Farmland Dairies Skim Plus or Ultra Skim Milk

65 Walden Farms Calorie-Free Chocolate Sauce

66 Oscar Mayer Fat-Free Hot Dogs

67 I Can't Believe It's Not Butter Spray

68 Jok 'n Al Fruit Spreads

69 Smart Dogs Tofu Pups

70 Arizona Diet Ice Tea

71 Kraft Fat-Free Mayonnaise

72 Gardenburger Crispy Nuggets

73 Wonder 100% Whole Wheat Bread

74 Babybel Light Cheese Wedges

75 Laura's Beef Meat Products (especially ground beef and lean roast)

76 Starkist Crabmeat

77 Trader Joe's Meatless Meatballs

78 Imagine Organic Free-Range Chicken Broth

79 Trader Joe's Gazpacho Soup

80 Trader Joe's Organic Chicken Broth (5 calories a serving)

81 Breakstone or Cabot's Fat-Free Sour Cream

82 Cascadian Farms Organic Mixed Veggies

Taste Is King Awards—Continued

83 VitaMuffin

84 Smart Water or Fruit H_2O

85 Promise's Ultra Fat-Free Margarine

86 Alpine Lace Reduced-Fat Cheddar Cheese

87 Alpine Lace Reduced-Fat Fresh Parmesan Grated Cheese

88 Sorrentino or Stella Reduced-Fat Ricotta Cheese

89 Superskim Milk (looks and tastes like whole milk)

90 Friendship 1% Low-Fat No-Salt-Added Cottage Cheese

91 Hormel Turkey Pepperoni

92 Prego No-Salt-Added Pasta Sauces

93 Celestial Seasonings Teas

94 Healthy Choice Cold Cuts

95 Healthy Choice Country Vegetable Soup

96 Health Valley Vegetable Soups

97 Campbell's Low Sodium Soups

98 Tabatchnick's Frozen Soups

99 Pritikin Vegetable or Chicken Broth

100 Health Valley Beef or Chicken Broth

101 Herb-Ox Low Sodium Beef or Chicken Broth

102 Smart Beat Mayonnaisse

103 Patisserie de France Giurees (frozen orange or lemon skin filled with sorbet)

104 Alouette Light Garlic & Herb Cheese Spread

105 CarbFit Chocolate Chip Cookies (for maintenance only)

106 Walden Farms Calorie-Free Balsamic Vinaigrette

107 Cascadian Farms Mixed Berries

108 Boursin Light Cheese Spread

109 CarbSolutions Shakes

110 Designer Protein Shakes

RECOMMENDED SEAFOOD

SPECIES	CALORIES	PROTEIN (G)	OMEGA-3S (G)	FAT (G)	SATURATED FAT (G)	%DV CALCIUM	SERVING SIZE
Cod, broiled	90	19	0.1	1	0	>2	3 oz
Flounder, baked	100	20	0.4	1	0	2	3 oz
Haddock, baked	90	20	0.2	1	0	4	3 oz
Halibut, broiled	120	22	0.4	2	0	5	3 oz
Lobster, broiled	100	20	0.1	1	0	5	3 oz
Orange roughy	70	16	n/a	1	0	>2	3 oz
Atlantic salmon/coho, baked	150	22	1.6	5	0	>2	3 oz
Alaska salmon/chum	135	23	0	4	1	n/a	3 oz
Alaska salmon/pink	130	22	0	4	0.5	n/a	3oz
Sockeye salmon, canned	110	13	0	7	1.5	n/a	¼ cup
Pink salmon, canned	90	12	0.9	5	1	n/a	¼ cup
Scallops, broiled	150	29	n/a	1	0	2	14 small
Shrimp, boiled	110	22	0.3	2	0	3	6 large
Sole, broiled	100	21	n/a	1	0	2	3 oz
Blue mussels, steamed	90	19	0.7	3.8	1	n/a	3 oz
Blue crab, steamed	90	19	0.4	1	0	9	3 oz
Clams, steamed	130	22	0.2	2	0	8	12 small
Oysters, steamed	120	12	0.7	4	1	8	12 medium

RECOMMENDED FRUITS

FRUIT	CALORIES	CARBS (G)	FIBER (G)	%DV CALCIUM	SERVING SIZE
Apple	80	22	5	n/a	1 medium
Banana	110	29	4	n/a	1 medium
Blackberries	70	18	8	4	1 cup
Blueberries	80	20	4	n/a	1 cup
Cantaloupe	100	23	2	4	½ medium
Grapefruit	60	16	6	2	½ medium
Honeydew	130	33	3	n/a	½ medium

RECOMMENDED FRUITS—CONTINUED

FRUIT	CALORIES	CARBS (G)	FIBER (G)	%DV CALCIUM	SERVING SIZE
Kiwifruit	50	12	2	4	1 medium
Kumquat	50	12	5	4	1 medium
Lemon	15	5	1	2	1 medium
Lime	20	7	2	n/a	1 medium
Mandarin orange	45	11	2	6	1 large
Orange	45	14	5	4	100g
Peach	40	11	2	n/a	1 medium
Pear	100	25	4	2	1 medium
Persimmon	30	8	n/a	n/a	1 medium
Plum	80	19	2	n/a	2 medium
Prickly pear	40	10	4	6	1 medium
Raspberries	60	14	8	2	1 cup
Strawberries	35	8	3	n/a	1 cup
Tangerine	50	15	3	4	1 medium
Tangelo	60	15	3	6	1 medium
Watermelon	80	27	2	2	2 cups

RECOMMENDED VEGETABLES

VEGETABLES	CALORIES	CARBS (G)	FIBER (G)	PROTEIN (G)	%DV CALCIUM	SERVING SIZE
Artichokes	60	13	7	4	6	1 medium
Asparagus	25	4	2	2	2	5 spears
Beets	35	8	2	1	n/a	1 medium
Bell pepper	30	8	2	1	2	1 medium
Bok choy	50	9	4	6	45	1 cup
Broccoli	25	5	3	3	4	2 spears
Brussels sprouts	40	9	4	3	4	5 medium
Green cabbage	60	12	5	2	10	2 cups
Red cabbage	50	12	4	3	10	2 cups
Carrots (raw)	35	8	2	1	2	1 medium
Cauliflower	35	7	7	3	2	1 cup
Celery	10	3	1	>1	4	1 cup

VEGETABLES	CALORIES	CARBS (G)	FIBER (G)	PROTEIN (G)	%DV CALCIUM	SERVING SIZE
Celery root	40	9	2	2	4	1 cup
Sweet corn	120	27	4	5	n/a	1 ear
Cucumber	45	9	3	3	6	1 medium
Eggplant	140	33	14	6	4	1 unpeeled
Endive	10	2	2	>1	n/a	
Fava beans	80	13	5	6	2	1 cup
Fennel	70	17	7	3	10	1 medium bulb
Garlic	10	2	>1	>1	n/a	2 cloves
Green beans	30	6	4	1	5	1 cup
Boston lettuce	20	4	2	2	6	1 head
Iceberg lettuce	45	9	3	3	6	½ head
Red/greenleaf lettuce	20	4	2	1	6	1 cup
Romaine lettuce	15	2	2	2	4	1 cup
Crimini mushrooms	10	2	0	1	n/a	½ cup
Shiitake mushrooms	25	5	1	2	n/a	1 cup
Red onion	40	9	2	1	2	1 medium
Potato	100	26	3	4	2	1 medium
Pumpkin	50	12	3	2	4	1 cup
Radish	5	1		>1	2	2 radishes
Savoy cabbage	20	4	2	1	2	1 cup
Spinach (cooked)	20	4	3	3	10	1 cup
Butternut squash	60	16	5	1	6	1 cup
Crookneck squash	20	4	2	>1	2	1 cup
Hubbard squash	40	9	3	2	2	1 cup
Sweet potato	130	33	4	2	2	1 medium
Tomato	35	9	2	2	2	1 medium
Turnip greens	25	6	3	2	20	1 cup
Watercress	5	>1	>1	>1	4	1 cup
Zucchini	45	9	4	4	4	1 large

RECOMMENDED DIET BARS

BRAND	CALORIES	FAT (G)	CARBS (G)	FIBER (G)	SUGAR (G)	SUGAR ALCOHOL (G)	PROTEIN (G)	%DAILY CALCIUM	SERVING SIZE
Power Bar									
ProteinPlus Sugar-Free Caramel Apple	180	4	20	1	0	9	16	25	1.69 oz
ProteinPlus Sugar-Free Mocha Almond	170	2.5	20	1	0	18	16	25	1.69 oz
Pria PowerBar	170	8	21	n/a	n/a	n/a	10		1.69 oz
Pria	110	3	17	3	10	n/a	5	30	0.98 oz
Pria CarbSelect Cookies 'n' Caramel	170	7	22	2	1	18	10	30	1.69 oz
EAS									
AdvantEdge	220	6	20	2	1	n/a	25	30	2.12 oz
Myoplex Lite	190	4	27	1	18	n/a	15	25	1.97 oz
SlimFast									
Meal Options	220	6	35	>1	19	n/a	8	30	1.97 oz
Meal Bar	220	6	33	2	26	n/a	8	35	1.97 oz
Succeed	120	3	18	n/a	0	15	6	25	1.12 oz
Clif Bar									
Energy Bar	250	5	45	5	21	n/a	10	25	2.4 oz
Luna Bar	180	4	29	2	15	n/a	10	35	1.69 oz
Luna Glow-Strawberry Caramel Sundae	140	7	15	n/a	n/a	n/a	8	15	1.2 oz
Carb Solutions									
Taste Sensations	230	10	16	>1	1	n/a	24	50	2.11 oz
Candy Bar	140	10	17	>1	0	14	3	0	1.06 oz
Carborite									
Pecan Cluster Bar	110	7	16	>1	0	14	1	2	1.02 oz
Carbwise									
Chocolate Smore Crunch	240	9	24	>1	1	n/a	20	25	2.12 oz

BRAND	CALORIES	FAT (G)	CARBS (G)	FIBER (G)	SUGAR (G)	SUGAR ALCOHOL (G)	PROTEIN (G)	%DAILY CALCIUM	SERVING SIZE
Atkins									
Balance	200	6	22	1	17	n/a	14	10	50g
Advantage	220	11	22	11	0	n/a	18	30	60g
Biochem									
Strive	190	8	25	<10	0	n/a	20	25	2.1 oz
Worldwide									
Pure Protein	190	4.5	18	0	7	n/a	20	15	1.76 oz
Zone Perfect									
Nutrition Bar	210	7	23	1	11	n/a	14	4	1.76 oz
Whole Foods—365									
Verve-Meal Replacement Bar									
Peanut Butter Crunch	240	3.8	41	3	25	n/a	12	25	2.4 oz
Natural Cocoa with Chocolate Chunks	240	5	41	5	31	n/a	10	30	2.4 oz
Chocolate Chip Peanut Crunch	265	5.8	41	3	25	n/a	12	25	2.4 oz
Everyday Nutrition Bar									
Honey Peanut	175	4.0	18	2	15	n/a	18	30	1.76 oz
Chocolate Raspberry	190	4.0	17	1	16	n/a	17	30	1.76 oz
Chocolate Fudge	172	3.5	17	1	16	n/a	17	30	1.76 oz
Whole Foods—365 Organic									
Ella Nutrition Bar									
Peanut Butter Chocolate	180	4.5	28	2	12	n/a	10	22	1.7 oz
Chocolate Pecan	180	4.5	28	2	12	n/a	10	22	1.7 oz
Meyer Lemon	170	2	29	2	12	n/a	10	22	1.7 oz
Huckleberry	170	2	29	2	12	n/a	10	22	1.7 oz

Resources

FOODS AND SUPPLIES

Advanced Health Systems
Distributed by the Robard Corporation
821 East Gate Drive
Mt. Lowell, NJ 08054
Phone: 800-346-4422
Web site: www.robard.com or
  www.foodsciences.com
Maker of Fiber Plus Iced Tea with Lemon (one packet=15 calories) and Fulfill Mixed Fruit Drink (one packet=20 calories). These two high-fiber, low-calorie beverages are great for killing your appetite.

Cheese Supply, Inc.
PO Box 515
Vashon, WA 98070
Phone: 866-724-3373
Web site: www.cheesesupply.com
This is a great online source for many hard-to-find cheese items, such as Laughing Cow Light Cheese.

Egg Cream America, Inc.
633 Skokie Boulevard, #205
Northbrook, IL 60062
Web site: www.getcreamed.com
E-mail: GetCreamed@aol.com
The manufacturer of great-tasting, low-calorie drinks, including Jeff's Diet Chocolate Soda. They ship anywhere in United States.

Fage Total Yogurt
FAGE Dairy Industry S. A.
35 Hermou Street-GR 144 52
  Metamorfossi
Athens, Greece
Phone: +30 210 28 92 555
Web Site: www.fage.gr/page/default.asp

FAGE USA Corp
2526 50th Street
Woodside, NY 11377
Phone: 718-204-5323
Web site: www.fageusa.com

Fresh Direct
(for residents of New York City)
Phone: 866-288-7374
Web site: www.freshdirect.com
You can order prime quality groceries, produce, meats, and fish online for delivery at low prices.

Gayle's Miracles-Perfect
Chocolate Truffles
Manufactured by Gorant
  Candies, Inc.
8301 Market Street
Youngstown, OH 44512
Phone: 800-572-4139 to order
Web site: www.activewellness.com
E-mail: gayle@gaylesmiracles.com

GG Scandinavian Bran
Crispbread
Produced by G. Gundersen Larvik AS
Box 033
3251 Larvik, Norway
Phone: 0047-337-81-740
Web site: www.ggnorway.no
Distributed by Cel-Ent, Inc.
PO Box 1173
Beaufort, SC 29901
Phone: 866-266-1014
Web site: www.brancrispbread.com
Fax: 843-524-9444

The Hain Celestial Group, Inc.
4600 Sleepytime Drive
Boulder, CO 80301
Phone: 800-434-4246
Web site: www.hain-celestial.com
The Hain Celestial Food Group, including ALBA Shakes, Health Valley Soups, and Imagine Organic Broths, makes some of the best-tasting, low-calorie foods.

Institute of Eating Management
4801 Woodway, Suite 300 West
Houston, TX 77056
Phone: 713-621-9339
Web site: www.eatingmanagement.com
E-mail: info@eatingmanagement.com
This is the best online source for Keith Klein's Sugar Blocker Gum.

Joseph's Lite Cookies
3700 J Street SE
Deming, NM 88030
Phone: 505-546-2839
Web site: www.josephslitecookies.com
E-mail: josephs@josephslitecookies.com
Manufacturer of low-calorie sugar- and fat-free cookies, and maple syrup (endorsed by the National Diabetes Outreach)

Knight's Light Gourmet Popcorn
Web site: www.knightspopcorn.com

Laura's Lean Beef Company
2285 Executive Drive, Suite 200
Lexington, KY 40505
Phone: 859-299-7707, 800-ITS-LEAN
Web site: www.laurasleanbeef.com

Misto Gourmet Olive Oil Sprayer
Phone: 888-645-7772
Web site: www.misto.com
An easy-to-use, refillable sprayer that allows you to control the amount of oil you put on your food. Available at specialty food stores nationwide.

Synergy Diet LLC
1840 East Locust Street
Pasadena, CA 91107
Phone: 877-877-1558
Web site: www.synergydiet.com
This may be the very best online supermarket for great-tasting, low-carbohydrate foods, drinks, and supplements.

Trader Joe's Grocery Store
Web site: www.traderjoes.com
Trader Joe's is a unique grocery store with more than 200 locations nationwide.

Van's International Foods
Van's Waffles
20318 Gramercy Place
Torrance, CA 90501
Phone: 310-320-8611
Web site: www.vansintl.com
E-mail: customerservice@vansintl.com

Vitalicious
303 Greenwich Street, Suite 2-L
New York, NY 10013
Phone: 877-VITA-877
Web site: www.vitalicious.com
Makers of the 100-calorie VitaMuffin

Walden Farms
Phone: 800-229-1706
Web site: www.waldenfarms.com
E-mail: info@waldenfarms.com

Whole Foods Market, Inc.
Research and Support Team
700 Lavaca Street, Suite 500
Austin, TX 78701
Phone: 512-477-4455
Web site: www.wholefoodsmarket.com

RECOMMENDED WEIGHT LOSS AND EXERCISE PROGRAMS

Weight Watchers
Web site: www.weightwatchers.com

Jenny Craig International
5770 Fleet Street
Carlsbad, CA 92008
Phone: 760-696-4000; 800-597-jenny
Web site: www.jennycraig.com

LA Weight Loss Centers
Phone: 800-331-4035
Web site: www.laweightloss.com
More than 650 locations nationwide

Ediet.com
3801 West Hillsboro Boulevard
Deerfield Beach, FL 33442
Phone: 800-265-6170
Web site: www.ediet.com

WebMD Weight Loss Clinic
Web site: www.webmd.com

Overeaters Anonymous
World Service Office
PO Box 44020
Rio Ranchero, NM 87174-4020
Phone: 505-891-2664
Web site: www.oa.org
E-mail: info@oa.org

Curves International Exercise Studio
Phone: 800-848-1096
Web site:
www.curvesinternational.com

RECOMMENDED BOOKS

Agatston, Arthur, M.D. *The South Beach Diet.* Emmaus, PA: Rodale, 2003.

Gullo, Stephen, Ph.D. *Thin Tastes Better.* New York: Clarkson Potter, 1995.

Jacobson, Michael F., Ph.D., and Hurley, Jayne, R.D. *Restaurant Confidential.* New York: Workman, 2002.

McGraw, Phil, Ph.D. *The Ultimate Weight Solution.* New York: The Free Press, 2003. This book is especially helpful for emotional eating.

Rolls, Barbara, Ph.D., and Barnett, Robert A. *The Volumetrics Weight-Control Plan.* New York: HarperCollins, 2000.

Shapiro, Robert M., D.O. *Picture Perfect Weight Loss.* Emmaus, PA: Rodale, 2002.

Simpoulos, Artemis P., M.D. *The Omega Diet.* New York: HarperCollins, 1998.

Willett, Walter C., M.D. *Eat, Drink and Be Healthy: The Harvard Medical School Guide to Healthy Eating.* New York: Simon & Schuster, 2001.

Zemel, Michael, Ph.D., and Gottlieb, Bill. *The Calcium Key: The Revolutionary Diet Discovery That Will Help You Lose Weight Faster.* Hoboken, NJ: John Wiley & Sons, 2003.

RECOMMENDED PUBLICATIONS

The health publications many of my clients read regularly.

Prevention Magazine
Phone: 610-967-8527
Web site: www.prevention.com

Nutrition Action Health Letter
Center for Science in the Public Interest
1875 Connecticut Avenue, NW
Suite 300
Washington, DC 20009
Phone: 202-332-9110
Web site: www.cspinet.org

Tufts University Health & Nutrition Newsletter
Subscription Department
PO Box 420235
Palm Coast, FL 32142-0235
Phone: 800-274-7581
Web site: www.healthletter.tufts.edu
Editorial Questions
10 High Street, Suite 706
Boston, MA 02110

Mayo Clinic Health Letter and Mayo Clinic Women's HealthSource
Phone: 800-526-7204
Web site: www.mayoclinic.com

NOTED HEALTH COLUMNISTS

The following are a list of health/wellness columnists whose work I admire and read regularly. I believe you would benefit from their insights and wisdom.

Jane Brody
The New York Times
www.nytimes.com

Jean Carper
USA Today Weekend
www.stopagingnow.com

Dennis Kelly
USA Today
dkelly@usatoday.com

Tara Parker-Pope
The Wall Street Journal
www.wsj.com

Index

Underscored page references indicate boxed text.